Qualitative Inquiry and the Politics of Research

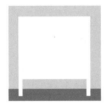

INTERNATIONAL CONGRESS OF QUALITATIVE INQUIRY

The International Congress of Qualitative Inquiry has been hosted each May since 2005 by the International Center for Qualitative Inquiry at the University of Illinois, Urbana-Champaign. This volume and the preceding ones are products of plenary sessions from these international congresses. All of these volumes are edited by Norman K. Denzin and Michael D. Giardina and are available from Left Coast Press, Inc. Main series volumes include

For more information on these publications, or to order, go to www.LCoastPress.com

Qualitative Inquiry and the Politics of Research

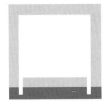

Norman K. Denzin & Michael D. Giardina

(Editors)

Walnut Creek, California

LEFT COAST PRESS, INC.
1630 North Main Street, #400
Walnut Creek, CA 94596
www.LCoastPress.com

Copyright © 2015 by Left Coast Press, Inc.

ISBN 978-1-62958-162-0 hardback
ISBN 978-1-62958-163-7 paperback
ISBN 978-1-62958-164-4 institutional eBook
ISBN 978-1-62958-165-1 consumer eBook

Library of Congress Cataloging-in-Publication Data:

Qualitative inquiry and the politics of research / edited by Norman K. Denzin & Michael D. Giardina.
  International Congress of Qualitative Inquiry (10th : 2014 : University of Illinois, Urbana-Champaign)
      pages cm. — (International Congress of Qualitative Inquiry ; 10)
  Includes bibliographical references and index.
  ISBN 978-1-62958-162-0 (hardback) — ISBN 978-1-62958-163-7 (paperback) — ISBN 978-1-62958-164-4 (institutional eBook) — ISBN 978-1-62958-165-1 (consumer eBook)
  1. Qualitative research—Congresses. 2. Interdisciplinary research—Congresses. 3. Research—Congresses. 4. Learning and scholarship—Congresses. I. Denzin, Norman K. II. Giardina, Michael D., 1976- III. Title.
  H62.I657 2014
  001.4'2—dc23
                        2015003710

Printed in the United States of America

⊗™ The paper used in this publication meets the minimum requirements of American National Standard for Information Sciences—Permanence of Paper for Printed Library Materials, ANSI/NISO Z39.48–1992.

Contents

In memoriam

Gregory J. Dimitriadis

Scholar. Educator. Friend.

Acknowledgments

We thank our publisher of all publishers, Mitch Allen, for his continued support and guidance throughout the years. We also thank Michael Jennings for expert copyediting, Hannah Jennings for fantastic production design, and Neal Ternes for assistance in gathering the index. Many of the chapters contained in this book were presented as plenary or keynote addresses at the Tenth International Congress of Qualitative Inquiry, held at the University of Illinois, Urbana-Champaign, in May 2014. We thank the Institute of Communications Research, the College of Media, and the International Institute for Qualitative Inquiry for continued support of the Congress as well as those campus units that contributed time, fund, and/or volunteers to the effort.

The Congress, and by extension this book, would not have materialized without the tireless efforts of Mary Blair, Katia Curbelo, Ted Faust, Bryce Henson, Shantel Martinez, Robin Price, Nathalie Tiberghien, and James Salvo (the glue who continues to hold the whole thing together). For information on future Congresses, please visit www.icqi.org.

Norman K. Denzin

Michael D. Giardina

December 2014

Introduction

Qualitative Inquiry and the Politics of Research

Norman K. Denzin and Michael D. Giardina

If the university does not take seriously and rigorously its role as a guardian of wider civic freedoms, as interrogator of more and more complex ethical problems, as servant and preserver of deeper democratic practices, then some other regime or ménage of regimes will do it for us, in spite of us and without us.
(Toni Morrison, 2008, p. 278)

Proem[1]

We begin with two headlines, appearing on back to back days, from January 27 and 28, 2015: "Walker Unveils $220 Million [Milwaukee] Bucks Arena Funding Plan" (Armas, 2015) and "Walker Proposes $300 Million Cut to University of Wisconsin System, New Freedoms" (WPRG.org, 2015). Read together, the Governor of Wisconsin was proposing a 13 percent cut in state funding for the University of Wisconsin system at the *exact same time* he was proposing a $220 million state-level investment in a new, state of the art downtown sports arena that would house, among other entities, the Milwaukee Bucks of the National

Qualitative Inquiry and the Politics of Research edited by Norman K. Denzin and Michael D. Giardina, 9–25. © 2015 Left Coast Press, Inc. All rights reserved.

Basketball Association; the billionaire owners of the team would contribute roughly $150 million to the project; all remaining funding would come from local counties and tax revenues. And this is what he calls a "common-sense, fiscally conservative approach" (Walker, 2015, para. 1).

The optics of the two announcements should not come as a surprise to anyone, nor should their ideological framing, twinned as they both are to the language of the free-market and its profound impacts on civil society. In the first instance, Walker stated that the proposed budget cuts would force the university system to "be more effective, more efficient," while also arguing that university professors should be "teaching more classes and doing more work" (quoted in McCalmont, 2015, paras. 6, 1). His statements should not be surprising; the focus on 'efficiency' and other such 'accountability metrics' and 'deliverables' has over the last decade become the new watchword of higher education (as have more baseless political attacks on teachers more generally). Who among us has not found ourself wading through hours of endless paperwork, annual reports, journal impact factors, student and peer evaluations, credit-hours generated matrices, and other measures that seek to quantify one's contribution to the university—what Yvonna S. Lincoln has termed "a neoliberal, managerial, technocratic set of means for regulating and normalizing behavior" (p. 370)? And who among us has not read articles in mainstream publications with titles such as "The War on Teacher Tenure" (Edwards, 2014), "Humanities Studies under Strain around the Globe" (Delaney, 2013), and "GOP Pushes Funding Cuts for Social Science Work" (Jan, 2014)? Yet what Walker and others of his mindset overlook (or choose to ignore) is that

> such trivial measures fail to take account of the extra-class teaching that goes on: the undergraduate advising; the doctoral dissertation consultations; the public service rendered to schools, civic organizations, business enterprises and even the Federal government; the internal governance and committee work; the student organization advising; the knowledge generation activities which are unfunded but critical to maintain our own cultural heritage; the administration—all of which enriches the

educational enterprise in countless, but primarily unremunerated, ways. (Lincoln, 2010, para. 5).

Beyond this crass devaluation of the role of the professoriate—a professoriate that has already been demoralized through previous budget cuts and university transformations—is that tucked neatly into Walker's proposed cuts is the reorganization of the university system in such a way that "would eliminate state laws governing the UW system" (Marley & Herzog, 2015, para. 24); two of those state laws currently govern faculty tenure and shared faculty governance—ideas that many would view as sacrosanct to the functioning of a university in any critical formation.[2]

In the second instance, the notion that a publicly funded sports arena would be an economic panacea is belied by decades of research on stadium and arena construction and funding projects (see, e.g., Noll & Zimbalist, 1997; Zirin, 2013). One need only look to the myriad examples in recent years to see this myth in action. For example, at the very same moment that Detroit, Michigan, was declaring its bankruptcy in 2013, Michigan's Republican Governor, Rick Snyder, was approving a plan for a brand new $650 million arena for the Detroit Red Wings of the National Hockey League, of which roughly half of the funding would be paid with public funds (see Zirin, 2013, para. 3). Situated in market terms of "investment in the future of Detroit," the new arena has been positioned as a saving grace for rehabilitating the local economy. But as scores of critics have rightly pointed out, sweetheart stadium and arena deals contribute little to the solution of urban hardship and local economic frailty. In fact, as Marvin Surkin pointed out in an interview with Dave Zirin (2013), publicly funded stadiums in the Detroit area (as elsewhere) are actually "part of the problem because stadiums don't address the central issues of falling population, falling tax base, declining wages, unemployment, and the underfunding of schools" (para. 7). By that he means that

> this kind of corporate welfare has over the last generation exacerbated Detroit's existing problems ... because it siphons money out of the city services—things like schools and hospitals—while

creating the very kinds of jobs that are the antithesis to those that once built Detroit into the third-largest city in the United States. No living wages. No job security. No tax base. Just spanking new stadiums for suburban sports fans, which Detroit residents will be able to enter only if they're selling foam novelty fingers. (Zirin, 2013, para. 8)[3]

And here is where the two issues are joined: both the proposed cuts to the University of Wisconsin system and the public subsidy of the new arena in Milwaukee are examples of free-market orthodoxy at its best—in other words, it's *supposed* to work this way. Put differently, these developments lay bare the complicated "symbiotic relation between commercial and public spaces and their private appropriation through consumption" (Harvey, 2003, p. 217) that has come to dominate the United States. And it is a vision of the future that is unsustainable given the current trajectory of modern life.

It is within this context that *Qualitative Inquiry and the Politics of Research* is situated.

On the Politics of Research in the Neoliberal State

Today we find ourselves deeply ensconced in a moment of neoliberal fundamentalism (often referred to as market fundamentalism), or a belief in which all social and economic problems can always and only be solved through a free market economy (i.e., deregulation of business and trade, a restriction if not abolishment of state intervention, etc.). As an economic governing formation, neoliberal ideologues throughout the 1980s (and into today) advocated for

> unbridled entrepreneurial freedom, free markets, free trade, a radically reduced state, and vigorously promoted consumerism. Deregulation, privatization, market forces, and consumer choice became the watchwords of neoliberal states as they extolled the virtues of economic globalization and sought to provide the appropriate institutional setting within which economic growth could be maintained and corporations could significantly increase rates of profit by generating increasing consumption of goods and services. (Smart, 2010, p. 19)[4]

The key economic critiques of neoliberalism offered by the likes of David Harvey (2007), Karl Polyani (1944/2001), Noam Chomsky (2011), Naomi Klein (2008), and Joseph Stiglitz (2003), to name but a few, have propelled us forward into thinking our way through the political economic imperatives of our age. And, due to the collective (though often competing and even conflicting) ideas offered by thinkers as diverse as Wendy Brown (2006), Michel Foucault (2008), Henry Giroux (2004), and Immanuel Wallerstein (2008), we have arrived at a point in time when we can look at neoliberalism beyond simply

> the consolidation of power in the hands of the few; it *also* aggressively attempts to break the power of unions, decouple income from productivity, subordinate the needs of society to the market, reduce civic education to job training, and render public services and amenities as unconscionable luxury. (Giroux, 2004, p. 249, italics added)

This is the singular guiding principle of neoliberalism in the United States (and elsewhere) today: *the reorientation of the individual away from the social welfare and well-being of the state and toward a pure free market in which the individual is (in theory) free to pursue his or her own ends with minimal state intervention.*

But consider the effects of such a reorientation on subjectivity.[5] As Foucault (2008) reminds us, subjectivity is not something that is given to or created independently by the individual, but rather is an effect of power, knowledge, and history. Subject to the market orientation of everyday life, the consumer-citizen is one whose neoliberal self is constructed through consumption choices, choices that in total reaffirm the conditions by which those very consumers' livelihoods are often destabilized. This "neoliberal subjectivity," as Liz Bondi (2005) has written, is largely regulated by market interests, born of the idealized "economic man" (or what Foucault and others have termed *Homo economicus*). It is in this vein that the self has become a projection of achievement in the hypercompetitive, individualized, ahistoricized market society. This is what Trent Hamman (2009) is talking about when he explains,

> Indeed the central aim of neoliberal governmentality is the strategic production of social conditions conducive to the constitution

of *Homo economicus* ... [in which] individuals are compelled to assume market-based values in all of their judgments and practices in order to amass sufficient quantities of "human capital" and thereby become "entrepreneurs of themselves." (p. 38)

It is in such a society, he continues, that "exploitation, domination, and every other form of social inequality is rendered invisible *as social* phenomena to the extent that each individual's social condition is judged as nothing other than the effect of his or her own choices and investments (Hamman, 2009, p. 43, emphasis in original). Success or failure is thus positioned as the inherent choice of the individual alone, extant of any structural conditions or barriers one might face, and certainly not the responsibility of the State to assist otherwise.

Numerous scholars have written at length about the commercialization and commodification of the university under such a governing philosophy, especially in terms of university branding, political debates over state and federal funding, and the transformation of education into a transactional practice borne of a consumerist ethos (see, e.g., Bok, 2003; Giroux, 2007; Tuchman, 2009; Twitchell, 2004). This shift we might recognize as the practice by which "students now in higher education have gone through a commodified, marketized, and stratified education system prior to their entry in higher education, which has inculcated this consumerist position and an instrumentalist approach to learning more generally (Canaan & Shumar, 2008, p. 7). Indeed, branded signifiers (e.g., McDonalds, Starbucks, Nike, etc.) abound in university campuses, buildings, and new 'research parks'; student fees and tuition dollars are increasingly used to subsidize exploding intercollegiate athletics budgets and university marketing campaigns in an effort to 'compete' with other universities for tuition dollars; and traditional on-campus housing options have been transformed into gleaming new apartment complexes. Yet, as Derek Bok (2003) has cautioned, although these commercial practices "may have become more obvious" in recent decades, "they are hardly a new phenomenon in American higher education" (a phenomenon that can be traced back at least to the early 1900s) (p. 2). What *has* changed, Bok posits—and what has amplified the current commercial portents—has been the confluence of a number of contextual factors in the last 30 years: system-wide financial cutbacks in educational spending at the state and federal level; a nationwide public embrace of "private enterprise and entrepreneurship" that legitimated such efforts; a "lack of clarity" about academic values and the role of the university; and, perhaps most importantly for Bok, "the rapid growth of money-making opportunities provided by a more technologically sophisticated, knowledge-based economy" (p. 15).

And here is where we as academics come in. For although the commodification of the university experience, in its individual iterations (i.e., Nike sponsorships, partnerships with credit card companies, exploding marketing budgets, etc.), is one that may trouble us in the abstract, what concerns us more are the unseen struggles heralded by a market sensibility in terms of struggles over the *commodification of knowledge* and the *marketization of science*. Here the conduct of research becomes policed by an array of forces that impinge upon and (re)direct the practice of scholarly inquiry: namely, scholarly journals, promotion and tenure committees, federal funding agencies (i.e., National Science Foundation, National Institutes of Health, etc.), Institutional Review Boards, bibliometrics, and university political structures. In other words, the context in which 'science' is being conducted, and through which knowledge is produced and consumed, is one that is heavily influenced by the prevailing neoliberal condition, a condition in which positivist rationality (i.e., 'Gold Standard' research) is privileged, and knowledge has become instrumentalized in the pursuit of external grant dollars and other forms of capital accumulation. Henry Giroux (1983), for one, relays the consequences for such a turn:

> The outcome of positivist rationality and its technocratic view of science represents a threat to the notion of subjectivity and critical thinking. The question of essence—the difference between the world as it is and as it could be—is reduced to the merely methodological task of collecting and classifying facts. In this schema, 'knowledge relates solely to what is, and to its recurrence' (Horkheimer, 1972). Questions regarding the genesis,

development, and normative nature of the conceptual systems that select, organize, and define facts appear to be outside the concern of positivist rationality. (p. 15)

That is, as Michael Giardina and Joshua Newman (2013) surmise, "if scientific inquiry is molded around market forces, then the generative potentialities of new knowledge formations in and around a topic of inquiry [are] thus limited to their totemic epistemologies and methods" (p. 704). Or, following Robert Zemsky (2003), when "market interests totally dominate colleges and universities, their role as public agencies significantly diminishes—as does their capacity to provide venues for the testing of new ideas and the agendas for public action" (p. B9).

Returning to Foucault, we should not overlook the effects of this new context on our subjectivity. For, as Bronwyn Davies and Eva B. Peterson (2005) remind us, "management techniques [governing intellectual professionalism] individualize performance. They require individuals to negotiate annual recognizable accounts of themselves as appropriate subjects, and to stage a performance of themselves as appropriate(d) subjects. The academic accomplishes him or herself, for the moment of that performance at least, *as* a neoliberal subject" (p. 81, emphasis in original; also cited in Sparkes, 2013, p. 5). To that end, we would do well to consider the politics of (our) research in relation to questions of *evidence* (e.g., "What do we mean by evidence?" "What constitutes 'good' evidence?" "What kinds of ideological work might the phrase 'evidence-based research' do?"), *knowledge* (e.g., "How is knowledge generated, constructed, and disseminated?" "In what ways might the notion of 'knowledge production/translation' serve to narrow, rather than broaden, our discussions of contemporary social issues?"), and *research practice(s)* (e.g., "What kinds of research practices are privileged?" "Which dimensions of the practice of research receive too little attention in the texts we produce?" and "Where do we as academics fit within this context in the present moment?" (see especially Giardina & Laurendeau, 2013, p. 238).

This is the charge our authors have taken up in the pages of *Qualitative Inquiry and the Politics of Research*. From the politics of publishing, to theorizing new ontologies, from thinking through narrative and praxis, to radically reimagining the act of schooling, the chapters that follow blaze a trail for finding our way outside of our present condition, to help us "shake off what we think we know in order to lend our imaginations to vibrant and sometimes agonistic spectrums of experience" (Butler, 2013, n.p.)

The Chapters

Qualitative Inquiry and the Politics of Research is comprised of ten chapters which, taken collectively, capture the current landscape of research practices and politics, debates and dialogues, agreements and disagreements. Mirka Koro-Ljungberg, Elliot P. Douglas, David Carlson, and David J. Therriault's chapter ("An Unfinished Dialogue about Problematizing Knowledge Production in the Peer Review Process") opens the volume, and highlights dilemmas in publication processes and peer reviewing when it comes to interdisciplinary research. More specifically, the authors argue that such processes are imbued with various forms of Foucaultian power relations and complex micropolitical struggles. Drawing from their diverse backgrounds (e.g., education, educational psychology, engineering, qualitative methodology), they endeavor through the use of multiple examples to "place in relief the ways and means of knowledge production that appear divorced of power relations."

In Chapter 2 ("Critical Qualitative Research in Global Neoliberalism"), Gaile S. Cannell and Yvonna S. Lincoln take up the work of Foucault and his deliberations on neoliberalism as an entry point through which to advocate for a "critical social science that radically researches power and possibilities for resistance(s) and generates critical counter actions on the ground." To do this, the authors delve into Foucault's *Society Must be Defended* (2003) and *The Birth of Biopolitics* (2008) (including critique of those works). Specifically, they discuss three major themes that relate to the conduct of research within an increasingly global neoliberal condition: (1) the neoliberal reconstruction/privileging/protection of an economics of competition; (2) homo entrepreneur (i.e., the individual, human body of enterprise); and (3) saturation so complete that ideology is not necessary and is made invisible. They conclude by presenting four directions for researchers as they navigate this neoliberal terrain within the corporate university.

In Chapter 3 ("Practices for the 'New' in the New Empiricisms, the New Materialisms, and Post Qualitative Inquiry"), Elizabeth Adams St. Pierre looks beyond the present to the 'coming after,' to what is 'new' in 'new' and 'post' work. Framing the discussion as one of ontology, she takes us through the work of Foucualt (especially *The Order of Things* and *The Archaeology of Knowledge*) and Deleuze and Guattari. At the same time, she critiques how and why such work that purports to be 'new' or 'post' often fails to escape the trappings of its previous master of conventional humanist inquiry. She concludes by offering a way forward in thinking our way through the new empirical, material, posthuman, post qualitative inquiry.

In Chapter 4 ("The Work of Thought and the Politics of Research"), Patti Lather continues the engagement with ontology and new materialism(s), arguing that what is 'new' here is "the ontological insistence on the weight of the material and a relational ontology that transverses binaries." Moving from Judith Butler to Karen Barad, Lather reviews the feminist orientation of this 'new' work, before moving into a discussion of a sport and schooling project that might take up such a post qualitative imaginary. She also addresses how art and sculpture—specifically the Cloud Gate sculpture in Chicago—can spur questions about becoming and in-betweenness.

In Chapter 5 ("Qualitative Data Analysis 2.0"), Uwe Flick ruminates on key challenges to conducting qualitative inquiry that is premised on societal relevance. These challenges include the trends to 'big data' and 'big research,' and the necessary political imperatives imbedded within such trends; conducting qualitative research across cultures and geographic divides (including language barriers); and how are data analyzed in the present moment (and, what do we mean by data in the first place). He concludes by pointing to several directions for future consideration in regard to the next iteration of data analysis.

In Chapter 6 ("Critical Autoethnography as Intersectional Praxis"), Bryant Keith Alexander attends to the notion of 'bleeding borders' and 'bleeding identities' as it relates to the conduct of a pedagogy of doing. To that end, he begins by presenting his own story in a borderless frame—an autoethnographic vignette into blackness, sexuality, and intercultural belonging. He then presents two examples of poetic autoethnography, an approach that serves as "a liquidity of emotion that fuses the politics of story and form." He concludes by arguing that the classroom can serve as a borderless frame through which to tell the stories of, and better understand, our intersectional lives.

In Chapter 7 ("Writing Myself into Winesburg, Ohio"), Laura Atkins writes herself into the 'history' of Sherwood Anderson's *Winesburg, Ohio*, connecting the Clyde of its imagination to the Clyde, Ohio, of the present day. More specifically, the author engages with narratives of the Whirlpool Corporation and its alleged environmental misconduct that may (or may not) have led to a public health crisis concerning childhood cancer in the area. Drawing from fieldwork that included 30 interviews with residents who lived within the boundaries of the cancer cluster, Atkins relays how various individuals provided their own forms of evidence to construct a particular 'truth of community' about what happened in Clyde, and how that complicated, complicit 'truth' frames understandings of Clyde in the popular imaginary of its local residents.

In Chapter 8 ("The Three Rs: Remembering, Revisiting, and Reworking"), Patrick J. Lewis focuses on how important 'the story' is to the truth of life's fictions (to steal a phrase from Trinh), especially as it relates to (the politics of) schooling and children. Drawing from but also extending Vygotsky's work on children's play, Lewis makes an impassioned call for the use of storytelling to be central to pedagogical praxis. In the process, he critiques and complicates the current practices of schooling, and suggests a way forward through 'reciprocal partnership' in learning.

In Chapter 9 ("Teaching Reflexivity in Qualitative Research"), Judith Preissle and Kathleen deMarrais impress upon us the need for reflexivity in our scholarly and professional endeavors. They begin by engaging with the concepts of reflexivity, recursivity, and reflectivity, and how those terms bleed into and through each other. They conclude by presenting six strategies for incorporating reflexivity into the research act and the act of being an intellectual.

In the Coda to the volume ("The Death of Data"), Norman K. Denzin asks the reader to imagine a world without data, a world without method, a world without a hegemonic politics of evidence, a world where no one counts, a world without end.

By Way of a Conclusion

Qualitative Inquiry and the Politics of Research marks the tenth volume in our series of books that have emanated from the International Congress of Qualitative Inquiry. Over the last ten years, our previous volumes have highlighted such pressing topics as ethics (2007), evidence (2008), social justice (2009), human rights (2010), and advocacy (2011), to name but a few. But perhaps the question of the politics of research is our most serious of all, for it encircles all of us—from early career PhD student to late-career Full Professor—*whether we like it or not*. In an unusually frank discussion of research politics in the contemporary university, Stephen R. Forrest, Vice President for Research at the University of Michigan (who is also a highly regarded scholar in the field of electrical engineering), stated the following:

> Nobody likes to put the words "politics" and "research" in the same sentence (as I just did). It seems to be an awkward mix of our conception of the "philistine" with the "pure". But, like it or not, all research is political with deep social and moral dimensions. We must face that apparent contradiction and deal with it head on if we are going to be successful researchers whose ultimate goal is to deepen our knowledge of the natural world and humankind, which will ultimately make our planet a more interesting and hospitable home. (2010, n.p.)

What we have presented in this Introduction, and what we hope you will take from the chapters that form this volume, is that the enterprise of higher education sits at an unsettled crossroads. Perhaps such critical reflection on its condition will spur us to exercise the kind of curiosity of which Foucault (1997) speaks, the kind that "evokes the care one takes of what exists and what might exist; a sharpened sense of reality, but one that is never immobilized before it; a readiness to find what surrounds us strange and odd; ...a lack of respect for the traditional hierarchies of what is important and fundamental" (p. 325).

We have a job to do; let's get to it.

Notes

1 The discussion of neoliberalism in this Introduction draws on and updates arguments in Giardina & Denzin, 2013, pp. 444–446. Reprinted by permission.

2 Such an attack on higher education is not the singular domain of Gov. Walker, however. In early 2015, The Board of Governors of the University of North Carolina, stacked with loyalists of Republican Gov. McCrory, moved to fire University of North Carolina president Tom Ross, despite all outward indications that Ross was a popular and successful university president (Pierce, 2015). At the same time, as Geary (2015) points out, the same Board of Governors has moved 34 research centers and institutes in its domain under scrutiny, primarily because they focus on poverty, social change, diversity, and civic engagement. In terms of our own institutions, we can point to the problematic *un*-hiring of Steven Salaita at the University of Illinois due to his extramural political speech on Twitter, and the politically complicated situation at Florida State University with regard to the process of hiring its new president, John Thrasher.

3 In the words of Steven Miles (2010), this "seductive vision of the city that is promoted as a means of reasserting the legitimacy of the post-industrial city is *fundamentally* incompatible with that city's lived reality (p. 164)—and not at all aimed at ameliorating the problems faced by those citizens who are increasingly viewed as "disposable": racial and ethnic minorities, the poor, and the disadvantaged (see Giroux, 2010). Rather, rejuvenation plans for Detroit (as with other downtown areas across the country) call for it to be turned into a playground for wealthy suburbanites who want to play and experience hermetically sealed cultural diversity without having to actually live among such diversity (see, for example, similar transformations taking place in Downtown Los Angeles).

4 And as political *force*, we can look to the 1980s, when British Prime Minister Margaret Thatcher referred to the "Washington Consensus" on free market orientations toward private property rights, corporate growth and sustainability, and social welfare by the slogan TINA or "There Is No Alternative" (see Wallerstein, 2008, p. 1).

5 This paragraph is drawn from Newman & Giardina, 2011, pp. 216–217. Adapted with permission of the authors.

References

Armas, G. C. (2015, January 28). Walker unveils $220M Bucks arena funding. *Green Bay Press-Gazette*. Retrieved January 29, 2015, from www.greenbaypressgazette.com/story/news/2015/01/27/milwaukee-bucks-arena-funding-plan-unveiled/22405649/

Bok, D. (2003). *Universities in the marketplace: The commercialization of higher education*. Princeton, NJ: Princeton University Press.

Bondi, L. (2005). Working the spaces of neoliberal subjectivity: Psychotherapeutic technologies, professionalism, and counseling. *Antipode, 37*(3), 497–524.

Brown, W. (2006). American nightmare: Neoliberalism, neoconservatism, and de-democratization. *Political Theory, 34*, 690–714.

Butler, J. (2013). Commencement address. Montreal: McGill University. [audio recording]. www.feelguide.com/2013/06/07/listen-to-philosopher-judith-butlers-mcgill-commencement-address-on-value-of-reading-humanities

Canaan, J., & Shumar, W. (2008). *Structure and agency in the neoliberal university*. New York: Routledge.

Chomsky, N. (2011). *Profit over people: Neoliberalism and global order*. New York: Seven Stories Press.

Davies, B., & Peterson, E. B. (2005). Neoliberal discourse in the academy: The forestalling of collective resistance. *Learning and Teaching in the Social Sciences, 2*, 77–98.

Delaney, E. (2013, December 1). Humanities studies under strain around the globe. *New York Times*. Retrieved from www.nytimes.com/2013/12/02/us/humanities-studies-under-strain-around-the-globe.html

Denzin, N. K., & Giardina, M. D. (Eds.). (2007). *Ethical futures in qualitative research: Decolonizing the politics of knowledge*. Walnut Creek, CA: Left Coast Press, Inc.

Denzin, N. K., & Giardina, M. D. (Eds.). (2008). *Qualitative inquiry and the politics of evidence*. Walnut Creek, CA: Left Coast Press, Inc..

Denzin, N. K., & Giardina, M. D. (Eds.). (2009). *Qualitative inquiry and social justice*. Walnut Creek, CA: Left Coast Press, Inc.

Denzin, N. K., & Giardina, M. D. (Eds.). (2010). *Qualitative inquiry and human rights*. Walnut Creek, CA: Left Coast Press, Inc.

Edwards, H. S. (2014, October 30). The war on teacher tenure. *Time*. Retrieved from time.com/3533556/the-war-on-teacher-tenure/

Forrest, S. R. (2010). The politics of research. *Office of the Vice President for Research, University of Michigan*. Retrieved from research.umich.edu/blog/2010/10/20/the-politics-of-research/

Foucault, M. (1997). The masked philosopher. In P. Rabinow (Ed.), *Ethics: Subjectivity and truth* (pp. 321–328). New York: The New Press.

Foucault, M. (2008). *The birth of biopolitics: Lectures at the Colleges de France, 1978–1979*. New York: PalgraveMacmillan.

Geary, B. (2015, January 21). Duke and UNC have lost their spine. Retrieved from www.indyweek.com/indyweek/duke-and-unc-have-lost-their-spine/ Content?oid=4322299

Giardina, M. D., & Denzin, N. K. (2013). Confronting neoliberalism: Toward a militant pedagogy of empowered citizenship. *Cultural Studies↔ Critical Methodologies, 13*(6), 443–451.

Giardina, M. D., & Laurendeau, J. (2013). Truth untold? Evidence, knowledge, and research practice(s). *Sociology of Sport Journal, 30*(4), 237–255.

Giardina, M. D., & Newman, J. I. (2013). The politics of research. In P. Leavy (Ed.), *The Oxford handbook of qualitative research* (pp. 699–723). New York: Oxford University Press.

Giroux, H. A. (1983). *Theory and resistance in education: A pedagogy for the opposition.* New York: Bergin & Garvey.

Giroux, H. A. (2004). *The terror of neoliberalism: Authoritarianism and the eclipse of democracy.* Boulder, CO: Paradigm.

Giroux, H. A. (2007). *The university in chains: Confronting the military–industrial complex.* Boulder, CO: Paradigm.

Giroux, H. A. (2010). *Youth in a suspect society: Democracy or disposability?* New York: PalgraveMacmillan.

Hamman, T. (2009). Neoliberalism, governmentality, and ethics. *Foucault Studies, 6*(1), 37–59.

Harvey, D. (2003). *Paris, capital of modernity.* New York: Routledge.

Harvey, D. (2007). *A brief history of neoliberalism.* New York: Oxford University Press.

Horkheimer, M. (1972). *Critical theory: Selected essays.* New York: Continuum.

Jan, T. (2014, April 14). GOP pushes funding cuts for social science work. *Boston Globe.* Retrieved from www.bostonglobe.com/news/nation/2014/04/14/gop-pushes-funding-cuts-for-social-science-work/5q4mMRROhWuwHaC46lW23N/story.html

Klein, N. (2008). *The shock doctrine: The rise of disaster capitalism.* New York: Picador.

Lincoln, Y. S. (2010). Accountability, Texas-style. *21ˢᵗ Century Scholar.* Retrieved January 12, 2015, from 21stcenturyscholar.org/2010/09/09/accountability-texas-style-by-yvonna-lincoln/

Lincoln, Y. S. (2011). "A well-regulated faculty. . . ": The coerciveness of accountability and other measures that abridge faculties' right to teach and research. *Cultural Studies ↔ Critical Methodologies, 11*(4), 369–372.

Marley, P., & Herzog, K. (2015, January 27). UW System predicts layoffs, no campus closings under budget. *Milwaukee Journal-Sentinel.* Retrieved January 29, 2015, from www.jsonline.com/news/state-politics/walker-proposes-300-million-cut-more-autonomy-for-uw-b99433799z1-289929831.html

McCalmont, , L. (2015, January 29). Scott Walker urges professors to work harder. *Politico.* Retrieved January 29, 2015, from ,www.politico.com/story/2015/01/scott-walker-higher-education-university-professors-114716.html

Miles, S. (2010). *Spaces for consumption.* Thousand Oaks, CA: Sage.

Morrison, T. (2008). How can values be taught in this university. *Michigan Quarterly Review* (Spring), 278.

Newman, J. I., & Giardina, M. D. (2011). *Sport, spectacle, and NASCAR Nation: Consumption and the cultural politics of neoliberalism.* New York: PalgraveMacmillan.

Noll, R. G., & Zimbalist, A. (Eds.) (1997). *Sports, jobs, and taxes: The economic impact of sports teams and stadiums.* Washington, DC: Brookings Institution Press.

Pierce, C. P. (2015). Art Pope's North Carolina: School's out. *Esquire.* Retrieved from www.esquire.com/blogs/politics/The_Pope_Of_North_Carolina

Polyani, K. (2001). *The great transformation: The political and economic origins of our time.* Boston, MA: Beacon. (Original work published 1944.)

Smart, B. (2010). *Consumer society: Critical issues & environmental consequences.* Thousand Oaks, CA: Sage.

Sparkes, A. C. (2013). Qualitative research in sport, exercise, and health in the era of neoliberalism, audit, and New Public Management: Understanding the conditions for the (im)possibilities of a new paradigm dialogue. *Qualitative Research in Sport, Exercise, and Health, 5*(3), 440–459.

Stiglitz, J. (2003). *Globalization and its discontents.* New York: W. W. Norton.

Tuchman, G. (2009). *Wannabe U: Inside the corporate university.* Chicago: University of Chicago Press.

Twitchell, J. (2004). *Branded nation: The marketing of Megachurch, College Inc., and Museumworld.* New York: Simon & Schuster.

Walker, D. (2015, January 27). Walker proposes investment of $220 million for Bucks arena. *Milwaukee Journal-Sentinel.* Retrieved January 28, 2015, from www.jsonline.com/news/statepolitics/walker-jock-tax-will-cover-220-million-for-new-bucks-arena-b99433734z1-289935421.html

Wallerstein, I. (2008). 2008: The demise of neoliberal globalization. *Monthly Review*. Retrieved from mrzine.monthlyreview.org/2008/wallerstein010208.html

WPRG.com. (2015, January 27). Walker proposed $300M cut to UW system, new freedoms. *Wisconsin Public Radio*. Retrieved January 29, 2015, from www.wpr.org/walker-proposes-300m-cut-uw-system-new-freedoms

Zemsky, R. (2003, May 30). Have we lost the 'public' in higher education? *The Chronicle of Higher Education*, B7–B9.

Zirin, D. (2013, July 29). On vultures and red wings: Billionaire gets new sports arena in bankrupt Detroit. *The Nation*. Retrieved January 27, 2015, from www.thenation.com/blog/175467/vultures-and-red-wings-billionaire-gets-new-sports-arena-bankrupt-detroit

Chapter 1

An Unfinished Dialogue about Problematizing Knowledge Production in the Peer Review Process[1]

Mirka Koro-Ljungberg, Elliot P. Douglas, David Carlson, and David J. Therriault

Law is not pacification, for beneath the law, war continues to rage in all the mechanisms of power, even in the most regular. War is the motor behind institutions and order. In the smallest of its cogs, peace is waging a secret war.

(Foucault, 2003, p. 50)

So, if a narrow claim to "expertise" allows one to operate machineries of domination, that person is also positioned to leak the secrets of the machine, even to calibrate its parts toward opposite functions.

(Caputo & Yount, 1993, p. 8)

For many qualitative researchers interdisciplinarity offers possibilities for wider distribution of knowledge, access to broader knowledge, and a network of collaborators and knowing subjects (Kotowski & Miller, 2010). Interdisciplinary research is important in today's society to address complex social problems, but scholars engaging in interdisciplinary research may face many complex challenges, including a variety of negotiations and normative,

Qualitative Inquiry and the Politics of Research edited by Norman K. Denzin and Michael D. Giardina, 27–50. © 2015 Left Coast Press, Inc. All rights reserved.

political decision making (see, e.g., Greckhamer et al., 2008; Lorenzetti & Ruthenford, 2012). One possible dilemma has to do with the publication processes and peer reviewing of articles, especially within scholarship that cuts across different contexts and disciplines (see, e.g., Langfeldt, 2006; Laudel, 2006).

The event of peer-reviewing is an important and vital part of producing research and academic life. Peer review is used by journals to guide what work is published and used by authors to improve their work. The peer review process is commonly used to judge manuscripts' acceptability and "serves as a filter to improve the quality of research" (Elsevier, n.d.). However, problems may occur when using traditional guidelines to review articles based on qualitative research. Alternatively, uncritical transfer of review standards across disciplines or from one discipline to the reviews of interdisciplinary papers and projects may create friction and resistance (see also Langfeldt, 2006). There is evidence that qualitative work, especially creative, innovative work, or scholarship that is viewed to push the limits of normative qualitative research practices, does not get published as often as other works for various reasons (see, e.g., Beddoes, 2014). One reason might be a lack of knowledge about qualitative epistemologies, sometimes causing the use of inappropriate standards for reviewing. Another reason might have to do with the strong focus of journals on 'traditional' non-qualitative styles which have different approaches and formats than qualitative work (see also Langfeldt, 2006; Schoenberg & McAuley, 2007).

Although the peer-review event and process as an institutionalized form appears to be objective and rational, this chapter illustrates that it is fraught with various forms of Foucaultian power relations. Thus, the purpose of this chapter is to illustrate from multiple perspectives the complexities of micropolitics associated with interdisciplinary projects namely in relation to peer review and publication processes. As the first quote above indicates, we take the stance that even claims of peace represent a strategic move in the overall battle among various forms of domination. All authors of this chapter are members in different discursive communities and take part in diverse political practices within academia. Even though each of us has (at least slightly) different reasons to engage in this project, all of us desire to disclose the secrets, unspoken, and the silenced in the peer-review process, most notably, the endemic struggle of forces in seemingly sanitized and transparent processes. The following "unfinished dialogue or *dialogue raw/brute*" illustrates our changing and uncertain subject positions while reflecting on the knowledge production in the peer review process. Our unfinished dialogue builds from multiplicities of inquiries and wonderings without totality—wonderings that link together and connect with other wonderings and events (events that are also at least partially unformed, irrational, yet forceful). Through dislodged structures, forgotten strategies, abolished policies, and dispersion of concepts and perspectives we document our reflections and sensed experiences. In addition, this dialogue reflects our desires to face uncertainty, rawness, and perspectival chaos by doing, engaging, collaborating, and reflecting without predetermination, rationalization, continuous purification, and 'cleaning' efforts (see also Koro-Ljungberg, Carlson, Tesar & Anderson, in press).

The interdisciplinary work exemplified in this manuscript brings together engineering, education, educational psychology, and qualitative methodology. All these disciplines have different journals, and somewhat varying standards, practices, and expectations. The following Foucaultian analysis highlights the exchanges between authors and editors (reviewers), strategically problematizing these exchanges. By engaging in this problematization we place a "given into a question, this transformation of a group of obstacles and difficulties into problems to which the diverse solutions will attempt to produce a response" (Foucault, in Rabinow, 1984, p. 389). The acceptance and subsequent rejection of the article (discussed as an example in this chapter) problematizes academic subject positions in two ways. First, editorialship and authorship become problematized in that it removes the veil of objectivity, disinterestedness, and "blind peer-review." This process, although heralded as a means to determine the truth and to establish truth of a discipline against falsehoods, is fraught with multiple forms of power. Hence, from a Foucaultian standpoint, knowledge is always/already established via multiple discourses and practices of power as an action upon an action and as a means to demarcate spaces for academic subjectivities and subjection positions to be produced and fashioned (Foucault, 1983). Second, the authors of this chapter, by disclosing the events around the publishing process, problematize, or place in relief, the ways and means of knowledge production that appear divorced from power relations. The peer-review process itself comes under close scrutiny when methods of power/knowledge become revealed. In short, the peer-review publishing process, the sine quo non of academic life, is both problematized and is highly problematic, or in Foucault's terms, "dangerous."

This chapter also illustrates how power/knowledge/ethics/resistance interact in the academic arena. The implications of this work are epistemological, methodological, and ethical. Epistemologically, the reader sees how knowledge is produced through an agonistic relationship among various discourses and power relations (e.g., disciplinary, juridical, pastoral, and sovereign). Disciplinary power seeks to render bodies docile through subtle means of surveillance techniques and spatial arrangements; juridical power seeks to determine outcomes based on rights and rules (or laws); pastoral power strives to save or preserve the purity of a flock (group, or body) in order to progress to a greater or better future; and finally, sovereign power adjudicates, mostly in overt ways, the "right to take life or let live" (Foucault, 1978, p. 136). The numerous assemblages of power formations in this particular situation reveal how various forms of power produce knowledge.

Methodologically, the reader witnesses how one might operationalize Foucault's notions of power/knowledge in a "real-world, empirical" situation. More important, Foucault's nominalistic stance regarding historical and present events reveals its value in moments such as these. As he argues, profound events that generate historical or present change occur in the everyday reversals of power relations and not necessarily major events such as revolutions or mass protests (Flynn, 2005; Kendall & Wickham, 2000). It is events, such as the one described later in this chapter, that redesign and reconstruct the shifting spaces of power/knowledge relations that spur or foster larger alterations to discursive spaces. It is subjugated knowledges and experiences such as the ones described in this chapter that foster modifications and transformations of social spaces. In regard to ethics, the reader may also see how relations of power/knowledge allure and encourage academic subjectivities that produce a scholarly body. One final point, from a Foucaultian stand-point, hierarchies exist, but they are often used as a ruse to disguise more subtle forms of power/knowledge at play in a given relationship. They tend to be strategies used to produce specific subject positions in a given context. This means that all individuals in a given agonistic, contentious relationship have multiple strategies to acquire advantage over another or to dictate the procedures of battle to obtain their objective (Foucault, 1983).

Ideological and methodological differences and hierarchies produce power and create discourses that constitute and circulate knowledge and produce knowing subjects. In this chapter we were interested in different objects of scholarship, rituals, and the 'right to speak' within normative practices of research and publication, and we describe the progression of events as they unfolded in the peer-review process. The emails between our research team and the editors became the object of scholarship that was examined through normative rituals of the blind peer-review process. Throughout this process we were constituted differently as subjects and objects, and our position as the authors became realized only under the conditions of the normative review process. For example, at first we were constituted as knowing subjects, and we had a right to speak and to be heard when sharing our scholarship and research findings during the initial editor's review. However, later we were silenced, and reviewers were allowed to speak. Interestingly, the editor legitimatized the voice of the late third reviewer and positioned that reviewer as the knowing subject, ultimately even more knowledgeable than the editor. The rituals associated with the peer review process generated knowledge that eventually overturned the editor's first favorable publication decision.

Foucault (1980) referred to the crisis of the universities as opportunities to multiply and reinforce institutions' power effects as centers of individuals who relate and constitute the academic system. Thus, we should also consider the institutional site that made the editor's decisions possible—the site that serves as a legitimate source and point of application (Foucault, 1972). This editor positioned himself as an ethnographic listener interested in engineering studies, especially practices of knowledge in service, and whose actions are aimed to work against normative practices. The institutional site, in this context, is known both for its college of engineering and departments of engineering education and of science and technology in society. Furthermore, Journal X (impact factor 0.5) juxtaposes contributions from distinct disciplinary and analytical perspectives to encourage authors and readers to look beyond familiar theoretical, topical, temporal, and geographical boundaries for insight and guidance. According to the journal's editorial statement, the diversity in the editorial staff and board is designed to map the diversity in the field and support its persistence. The heterogeneity of perspectives in Journal X is its lifeblood, and the goal is high quality scholarship in every case. By these words Journal X marks its diversity, its democratic and justice oriented authority to regulate truth (science) and make distinctions between true and false, good and bad quality (of reviews and manuscripts).

In the following we discuss the events that constitute the micropolitics of this particular review process. To show how power operates as a network, we highlighted the most important forms of power working throughout the interactions between the authors and the journal editor. The dominate form of power in the interaction appears in all capital letters (e.g., JUDICIO), while the less important form of power appears in lower case letters (e.g., pastoral). This nomenclature is meant to be illustrative rather than psychological. We do not pretend to know the editor's intentionality in the exchange with the authors, and we do not claim a certain consciousness of the subjects involved in this process. We simply want to show how power produces knowledge and that power/knowledge operates within a network of forces. Finally, we put our examples of the different types of Foucaultian power in the text in proper order to offer the reader examples of these forms.

Events and Reflections

Event 1: Formal acceptance

Strategies: announcement of acceptance, establishment of formality of the review process [JUDICIO-disciplinary]

Editor x: As Editor of Journal X, I am delighted to formally accept your manuscript Discourses and engineering students' identities in engineering education and practice for publication in the journal.

The additional material you included in this draft helps considerably with the concern I raised earlier. Our next formal step is detailed below.

Event 2: Suspension of manuscript processing [judicio-PASTORAL]

Strategies: indication of worry and seriousness, self-disclosure and emphasis on past failure to notice the problems with the manuscript, publicity of record keeping, meditated decision making (weighing in options, increased legitimacy)

Editor x: Last week I received a late review of the revision you submitted *January 15*. A copy of it is below. As you know, I have kept the review of revisions in-house among associate editors, who have full access to the file.

The review concerned me greatly. It repeats three serious concerns that were raised by reviewers for the initial manuscript. I failed to emphasize the first in the summary portion of the August decision, although you acknowledged it in submitting the revision. The August decision summary did elaborate the second and third concerns. The December decision summary elaborated the second concern but not the third.

After pondering the case for several days, I am writing to let you know I must suspend the processing of this manuscript, pending your response to this review and letter. This step is unusual and unprecedented for me. Since it also potentially raises questions about my handling of the manuscript as Editor, I am informing my three fellow co-organizers of Network X, as well as the publisher. Should a subsequent decision alter the January acceptance, I want to be sure you have an avenue to appeal to the leadership. I would recuse myself from any deliberations of the co-organizers and abide by their decision.

Once again, the purpose of this letter is to alert you I had suspended processing this manuscript, pending your responses to these concerns [judicial]. I regret not having R3's review in time for the January decision. Since my primary responsibility is to ensure that all articles published in Journal X meet a minimum standard of quality, I am bound to take this step [pastoral].

Reviewer #3:
This paper has serious methodological and analytical problems that make me doubt the usefulness or value of the findings. I do not believe they are problems that can be fixed with a revision and I would recommend a decision to reject this article.

Event 3: Response to the suspension

Strategies: expression of dissatisfaction and unfairness, indication of authorship experience, questioning editor's ethics and decision making, response to the reviewers' comments [JUDICIO-disciplinary]

Submitting authors: We were quite disturbed to receive an email from the editor informing us that he has rescinded the acceptance of our paper and suspended its processing for publication [judicial]. Among the authors we have considerable editorial experience, and we have never encountered such a situation. Rescinding an article that has already been accepted is generally reserved for cases of clear fraud, such as fabrication of data or plagiarism. While this decision raises serious questions with respect to the process, for now we set aside those ethical issues to focus on the substance of the editor's comments.

Before addressing each of the specific points raised by the reviewer, we would like to address two general issues. First, the editor acknowledges his lack of knowledge in Discourse analysis, but then proceeds to accept the view of a single reviewer [disciplinary]. We would expect the editor to consult a diversity of sources in order to obtain a full understanding of a subject with which he might be unfamiliar. We question what privileges this particular reviewer's perspective over ours and other reviewers' who have supported the research. In fact, as we discuss below, the reviewer appears to have somewhat limited understanding of Discourse analysis.

David C.: From Foucault's perspective power is not possessed by anyone but it is always a network. I see in following examples nuances of power; pastoral power, sovereign power, and disciplinary power. Power is always influenced by knowledge and we can think about power as forces and action upon action. Power can also set up a space where certain relations can happen. In this paper I see pastoral power when one thinks that I need to preserve purity or integrity of this journal, field, or knowledge. The ways in which individuals do that they induce or lure the flock, namely writers and authors, to produce themselves in certain ways, and this is being done through different rhetorical ruses (see below). In this dialogue one can see some exemplary strategies to get the authors in line with what the journal or editor wants. Sovereign power is more overt form of power than we commonly see and get offended with; direct form of power where your boss tells you what to do. Sovereign power might function or be perceived as the least effective form of power since many people reject it. However, there are moments of sovereign power in these examples as well. Then, disciplinary power becomes visible in terms of

surveillance and many covert ways to govern and poten-
tially control people. In this moment of problematization and
(publication) crisis we need to think more thoroughly what it
means to be a scholar in Academia. This paper highlights many
micro physics of power and relational responses, the action upon
action that scholars can take when they are being encouraged to
produce certain scholarly body. I think we should also address
the macro physics of power; the institutional level (Caputo &
Yount, 1993; Foucault, 1983; Foucault, 1978).

Elliot: As a deputy editor of an engineering education
journal I try very hard to weigh what reviewers and associate editors say and how they say things. I also consider
what I know and what is important, especially when I get
conflicting reviews. For example, I could say in my editor's
letter, that I am not concerned about reviewer 2's comment on the small number of participants. Now looking
back into our experience I see that this editor abrogated
those responsibilities. He was simply going straight with
"oh this is what this reviewer said therefore I must follow
what the reviewer said." Even without considering the
fact that this happened after he accepted the paper which
put whole another layer onto it. Even if the third review
would have come in earlier the way in which the editor
responded abrogated that critical and reflective responsibility that an editor has to weigh what reviewers say and
help authors to understand what is important and not.

David C.: The editor employed pastoral strategies to get
his way to have the paper rejected, modified, or whatever.
He employs certain strategies to make sure that happens.
These strategies call for relational response from others
involved as to what does it means to produce knowledge
in Academia and who gets to say those things. Some
people are employing these strategies whether pastoral,
sovereign, disciplinary, or biopolitical, sometimes more
than one at the same time. These people are afforded by
different discourses to negotiate knowledge and epistemologies. It is possible the people employing pastoral

strategies misguided inappropriately are not 'caught' since they are feared and it is their responsibility to take care of the flock. It could be interpreted that this editor did not employ very good pastoral power since he was in some ways getting caught due to the position that all the writers are in; they don't need the publication per se and as such the authors have opportunity to respond back multiple ways in the power relationship.

Elliot: It was also interesting that the editor insisted that he was not rescinding the acceptance of the paper; he was only suspending the publication process. To me he was trying to rationalize to himself what he was doing by smoothing out what his actions meant.

David T.: The editor reached out to his constituents to check out if this [his actions] was okay or not. And those constituents then reported that there is no problem here. These actions also broke the blind review process by involving other people in the process and decision making outside blind reviewers. Without checking if this process was okay with us. We had double jeopardy. We were charged for some horrible editorial crime twice.

David C.: This is typical, this double jeopardy this trial. His (the editor's) strategy to send the manuscript out to two new reviewers and I check with my group to see if I am legal and following the responsibilities of my role. Using multiple forms of power to manipulate and get what one wants.

Event 4: Adjudication

Strategies: creation of fair hearing, establishment of 'external' review committee [JUDICIO-pastoral]

Editor: Thank you for your detailed reply to my March 12 message. I'm writing now for two reasons. The first is to say I have not rescinded the acceptance of your manuscript [pastoral]. I have, however, suspended its processing pending a review and final adjudication of the case. Your reply is part of that review. Secondly, as I indicated in my previous message, I have alerted both the organizers and the publisher of the action I was taking to suspend processing [judicial]. The publishing contract is with Network X, and the entire editorial staff serves at the pleasure of that organization. Since my action is both unusual and unprecedented, Network X organizers are establishing an ad hoc committee to review the case and make a recommendation for further action. Technically, the review committee is advisory to me, since only the editor has final authority in publishing decisions. However, as I also indicated in my message,   I will abide by their recommendation. The review committee consists of five prominent scholars and includes considerable expertise relating to the substantive contents of your study.

Event 5: Inquiry about the timelines

Strategies: creation of acceptable timeline, resistance to external decision making (judicio-PASTORAL)

Submitting authors: Thank you for your email. As you know the manuscript has been under review for quite some time. Several of the co-authors are junior scholars and timely publication of this paper is important for their careers [pastoral]. We do not want there to be any unnecessary delays and believe that two weeks should be sufficient for the committee to render its decision. We look forward to receiving the committee's response [judicial].

Mirka: We were guilty of analytical fraud.

Literature: Qualitative research is context and discipline based, and therefore consensus related to the quality of qualitative research is challenging and potentially not even desirable (Koro-Ljungberg, 2010; Taylor, Beck, & Ainsworth, 2001). Rolf quoted in Crescentini and Mainardi (2009) states that "any attempt to establish a consensus on quality criteria for qualitative research is unlikely to succeed for the simple reason that there is no unified body of theory, methodology or method that can be collectively described as qualitative research..." (p. 431). Nevertheless, various authors have addressed validity and established guidelines for reporting of qualitative research (e.g., Bowen, 2010; Duran et al., 2006; Lather, 1994; Maxwell, 2010; Scheurich, 1996; Taylor, et al., 2001; Zaruba et al., 1996; Wolcott, 1990). For example, the Standards for Reporting on Empirical Social Science Research in AERA Publications provides a guide for rigorous and ethical research while it also mentions that certain types of research will digress from the listed criteria (Duran et al., 2006). A general summary of the criteria in this guideline includes: formulation of problem; logic and design of inquiry; sources of evidence; measurement and classification; analysis and interpretation; generalization; and ethics (Duran et al., 2006). Similarly, Zaruba, Toma, and Stark (1996) proposed seven main categories for solid educational qualitative work: writing and focus, topic and audience, background and purpose, sampling, research methods, term definition, and presentation of findings/conclusion whereas Taylor et al. (2001) discussed qualitative researchers' desire for a descriptive sample, explanation of limitations, thick descriptive data, and how qualitative inquiry can contribute to knowledge.

Elliot: That's an interesting consideration, the tension as editor between being a "gatekeeper" of quality and a guide to help authors. When I make decisions on manuscripts I do try to give constructive advice on how authors can improve their manuscripts, even if the decision is not to publish. In this case we are only guessing. The editor admitted that he is not expert in discourse analysis. We don't know who the third reviewer was but the editor at least believed that this reviewer was an expert in discourse analysis and therefore gave precedence for this person's views over himself and other two reviewers. Maybe the editor got a feeling of "I screwed up."

David C.: These events problematize the peer review process in multiple ways. If you are to subject authors to double jeopardy and put them into this legalistic bind where they have to question if they want to publish in that journal or not. Or whether the work they have done is valuable or not. This calls into question what are the rights of the authors in the review process. It is also interesting to think that if the editor is not going to obey legalistic and existing practices and rules for any reason and he is going to employ pastoral and disciplinary power because he cannot do it through legalistic practices then the rules of the authors should shift too.

Event 6: Call for additional reviews

Strategies: relinquishing decision making power to external committee, meditated decision making (weighing in options, increased legitimacy), establishment of consensus and agreement, reference to the obligation and duty, support of (un)ethical conduct, re-review by the same reviewers who had 'serious concerns' earlier, support to sound review process, possibility of potential editorial changes in the future (not affecting this case) [JUDICIO-disciplinary]

Editor x: The Ad hoc Editorial Review Committee of *xxx Journal* has come up with recommendations after long deliberation regarding the manuscript, "Discourses and engineering students' identities in engineering education and practice." We addressed a number of questions as per our charge, and are in full consensus about the following findings: We agree that it is appropriate for the Journal's Editor to suspend a manuscript following an "accept" decision if he or she believes there is sufficient reason to warrant such action [judicial]. The editors and editorial board of the journal have an obligation to preserve the reputation and quality of the journal [pastoral]. However, there are also obligations to the author once a manuscript is accepted [judicial].

Conditions for the subsequent rejection of the manuscript should be based only on quite stringent criteria consisting of fraud or significant error, including errors of fact, misapplication of theory, or improper study design. Once a manuscript has been accepted, a decision to rescind acceptance must be based on no reason other than the merit of the paper or the actions of the authors. There should also be due process in reaching such a decision, although the decision whether to reject the manuscript or request further revisions should continue to rest with the editorial review process.

In the case of this manuscript, we find that there are sufficient concerns with this manuscript to warrant further editorial review. The authors are right to assert that a single review received from an associate editor should not be the basis for rejecting the manuscript (it is appropriate to suspend processing of a manuscript on this basis). Nor is this ad hoc committee the appropriate body to make such a decision. To ensure due process, we recommend the following:

- The manuscript should be sent out to two reviewers. One of the reviewers should be the second reviewer (R2) in the original review. The other should go to a scholar familiar with Gee's theory of discourse analysis and with appropriate standards for qualitative research [disciplinary].
- In fairness to the author, the scope of the review should be limited to the specific issues brought up by Reviewer 2.

We do regard the overall editorial process of the Journal to be sound. However, we believe there are some minor changes to the editorial process that would reduce the likelihood of a similar situation occurring in the future. Some of the existing procedures may in fact have been misleading to the authors, and may have caused additional work. We regard this to be an internal matter that will be addressed separately by the Editorial Board and suggest this document be transmitted directly to the authors.

Event 7: Withdrawal of the paper

Strategies: expression of disappointment, disengagement, concerns about ethical implications for future authors, reconstituting authors' expertise and choice of the publication outlet [disciplinary-PASTORAL]

Submitting authors: Thank you for completing the Ad Hoc process. As a result of you not standing behind your original decision to accept the paper but send it for another round of reviews by the very same person who initially disagreed with our interpretation of Gee's analysis we withdraw our paper. We would also like to express our deep disappointment regarding how our reviews were handled. The editor did not select reviewers who were appropriately familiar with Discourse analysis and interpretive research, inappropriately lengthened the review process by attempting to shape our paper to fit his own conceptions, and did not follow ethical principles for editors [disciplinary]. We worry about the ethical implications your decision potentially has to other scholars submitting to this journal [pastoral]. In addition, the editor's unexpected phone call to the lead author was rather odd and inappropriate. His tone was that of a teacher instructing a novice student about how the review process works. Further, his statement during the conversation that we did not apply Gee's theoretical structures appropriately makes it clear that further review by this journal would be quite pointless. It would have been much better if the editor had rejected the manuscript earlier if this is what he believed [disciplinary]. As it is we have spent more than a year and half in this process; time that could have been spent working with a different journal.

David C.: Juridical and legalistic issues here are interesting. The editor tried to force the authors to be scholars in a certain way but he was also pursuing these juridical types of power that are easily manipulated and he can work behind the scenes. I think it would be interesting as a response to these kinds of issues to come up with a yelp page for journals and people's experiences with the journals. This way the journals would need to become more responsible and accountable. My guess is that this type of thing happens a lot behind the scenes and I have heard many similar stories. Action upon action and using social media as a response and authors will fight back. If we were junior scholars this would be a huge deal for tenure and jobs and so on.

Mirka: I would like to return to ethics; people's capabilities to meet the other and unknown and how to respond when the path is not given. What do we do? This editor responded and followed his duty to promote rigorous scholarship but stumbled in how to meet the unknown and what to do in unexpected situations.

David T.: We signed a form that we will not submit this paper to another journal thus committing to this journal but the journal never committed to us. What if we would have decided to submit to another journal after they stopped processing our manuscript? Would that had been unethical behavior?

Elliot: Interesting you say that. My brother is a law professor and he told me that the way you publish articles in law journals is you do send it out to multiple law journals (each law school has their own journal) and you wait for offers. And if you get an offer from less prestigious journals and you are still waiting to hear back from more prestigious journals you tell the other journals to expedite their review so you can decide which journal to publish in (J. A. Douglas, personal communication, November 14, 2014). This practice clearly shifts the power relationships compared to how publishing occurs in education, science, and engineering journals. Rather than

*serving a gatekeeper role, it seems to me that in the law jour-
nal practice editors could become something like a stockbroker,
trying to get the best portfolio. So I wonder what would have
happened with our article under that model. Would the editor
have been more willing to "forgive" what he thought were
errors?*

*David C: From Foucault's standpoint when due processes
and considerations of the contract have been breached then it
becomes a matter of strategies. Ethics becomes a way in which
strategies are being employed and negotiated; action upon
action. The editor's ethical practices can be also a way to cover
up ethics that he violated. Many of these unethical practices
are never talked about and then they become subjugated
knowledges.*

Peace Waging War and Institutional Leakages

According to Foucault et al. (1991) power is exercised within
shifting discourses, and power is often expressed and represented
as an effect of strategic positions. For example, the strategic position of an editor enabled him to overturn his initial decision and
rely solely on the recommendations of the third reviewer. Power
produced knowledge; a reviewer was viewed as knowledgeable
and a knowing subject. The editor constituted himself and the
authors in relation to the third reviewer, peers, home institution,
field of study, other reviewers, our text, and the study. A part of
the docile body of the authors is also linked to the notion of time.
Editors control time, create time, and forget time. Docile authors
wait patiently.

Power is exercised through actions and various mechanisms
(e.g., examination and documentation) (Foucault, 1980). For
example, the role of examination provides another interesting
reflection point here. According to Foucault et al. (1991) examination combines techniques of observing hierarchy and normalizing judgment. Editors and reviewers are privileged due to the
hierarchy established by publishers and professional organizations to review authors' papers, whereas normalizing judgment

allows qualifications and classification. Manuscripts are qualified as strong or weak and thus classified as publishable or unpublishable. Rituals of examination are highly organized to guarantee and establish truth. Rituals of submission, including cover letter, styles, disclosure of conflicts of interest, are followed by the rituals of reviewing, including detailed and critical reviewer letters, anonymity of the reviewers, revision requests, invitations to revise and resubmit, and citation requests, among others. Yet, only some of these rituals and mechanisms are visible to or disclosed to the subjects. Foucault et al. (1991) wrote that "in discipline, it is the subjects who have to be seen. Their visibility assures the hold of the power that is exercised over them" (p. 187). Those whose work is to be examined experience or witness not the direct power but the effects of (anonymous) power. Knowledge of the privileged is transformed into a political and financial investment. Articles (both accepted and rejected) are political investments and discursive practices.

The examination (peer review) is followed by documentation and judgment (the letter of acceptance or rejection). Documentation makes the effect of power permanent and final. Through documentation the authors have been formalized as objects within the system of publication and peer review. As our example illustrates, our submission became a case that needed to be dealt with. Our case was forwarded to the legitimized members of the editorial board for further 'independent and unbiased' reviews. The editorial board members agreed with the editor's interpretation and legitimized his decision to overturn his original publication decision. Existing mechanisms supported existing hierarchy.

The events described in this chapter also reveal how power relations inform knowledge production. Problematizing the peer-review process, which is often seen as a clean process, offers insight into the various mechanisms that move in and through a key aspect of academic life. Experts conditioned by and beholden to the publishing "machineries of domination" also "leak the secrets of the machine" (Caputo & Yount, 1993, p. 8). Event 1 shows that the manuscript was originally accepted for publication, which, from a historical and traditional point of view, indicates that, pending minor emendations, the paper was to be published in the journal. The authors disciplined themselves and the knowledge to meet the standards of the journal, and after close scrutiny from peers exhibiting pastoral care, their work was "accepted" into the larger field of scholarship. Their word, from a pastoral care standpoint, reflected and exhibited the necessary purity to be deemed worthy to be part of the "flock" of knowledge. From a juridical standpoint, the administrative processes of submitting and fulfilling the necessary tasks to go under a peer-review process, their rights were not violated. In most cases, the manuscript would be published in the journal. The peer-review process becomes problematized in Event 2 when the manuscript is suspended. The subsequent events illustrate how peace wages war and how experts leak the secrets of their own institutions.

In this event, the editor of the journal employed a juridico-pastoral power. Juridical in the sense that he decided to pull the manuscript from the publication process, in short not allowing it to live, and he also informed the authors of their rights in the event that the article is ultimately rejected ("I want you be sure you have an avenue to appeal to the leadership"). Pastoral care appears when he claimed that the primary responsibility is to "ensure that all articles published in Journal X meet a minimum standard of quality, I am bound to take this step." Besides the fact that the editor withdrew the original acceptance from the manuscript, more important is that he shifted the rules of the publishing process. The editor decided to include a third reviewer's comments after notifying the authors the paper was accepted for publication. Although the editor changed the rules in his favor, couched in pastoral power to preserve the sanctity of the journal (e.g., knowledge), he failed to offer an equal shift in power relations on behalf of the authors. What this might look like is revealing the identity or the qualifications of the third reviewer. The authors believed they had employed Gee's discourse analysis properly; how would they know the third reviewer had any experience with Gee's methodologies? More specifically, rather than employ the juridical power of the "appeal" to an editorial board, why not simply equalize power relations using the same pastoral care that the editor administers.

To preserve the sanctity of knowledge, the third reviewer and the authors could have engaged in a fruitful exchange that could have potentially aided the authors in their revisions, preserved scholarship, and maintained the integrity of the journal. In fact, in event three, the authors spoke to pastoral power when they implored the editor to consult a diversity of experts to review the manuscripts methodology section. Instead, the editor leaned toward judicial and sovereign power, put the paper on life-support, yet refused to pull the plug on it. Instead, he and the review panel (see events 5 and 6) established a space for others (e.g., authors, editorial board), the "right to take life or let live" (Foucault, 1978, p. 136). Furthermore, as all those involved changed the rules of game, they neglected to alter them on behalf of the authors. Full disclosure of the review panel's meeting would have offered more transparency to the authors. The editor, in a strategic move, veiled as pastoral power, demarcated a space for the paper to die in an attempt to sacrifice the integrity of the journal and the peer-review process. Power relations, in this case, dominated knowledge production.

The previous dialogue also illustrates the shifting power relationships throughout the peer-review process and who counts as a knower. Initially, the authors were the knowers who collected the data, analyzed it, and framed the findings within an appropriate context. However, once they submitted the manuscript, power shifted to the editor. His decisions as to who were credible reviewers defined both him and the reviewers as the competent knowers with authority to judge the worthiness of the paper. As discussed by Frank (2013), this is a form of testimonial injustice. What is defined as quality becomes reified through the normative practices of a particular journal. Frank states that "journal editors do their best to ensure that every paper submitted to a journal receives a fair and unbiased hearing" (p. 366), and attributes the rejection of quality manuscripts to "difficulties" with the review process. It is possible that the editor may have difficulty finding reviewers who can fairly review particular methodologies or research approaches. However, such "difficulties" go beyond procedural issues and instead represent those normative practices that serve to consolidate and maintain power in the hands of the editor and editorial board. Journal review practices are sometimes reflective of a particular epistemology, which in turn serves to control knowledge and power (Kasman, 2003). Interestingly, in this case the editor appeared to relinquish his power by appointing a review panel to re-consider his decision. But in fact because the panel was appointed by him and chaired by a member of the journal's editorial board, it was not even possible for this panel to consider and judge or evaluate in ways different from the journal's accepted ways of knowing and practicing. As discussed by Frank (2013), when we limit who we see as a competent knower we bound our ability to gain a full understanding of our complex world and experiences. In addition, by narrowly defining what counts as "truth" or by using the "right method" as the fixed standard, scholarly communities might severely bound their ability to see diverse perspectives and support diversified and less familiar practices. 'Strange and foreign' in methodologies could be welcomed and negotiated rather than placed under immediate normalized judgment. Maybe we hesitantly title our learnings and dialogue as "An Unfinished Dialogue about Problematizing Knowledge Production in the Peer Review Process."

Note

1 We would like to thank Amy Bumbaco for her assistance in preparing the literature review.

References

Beddoes, K. (2014). Using peer reviews to examine micropolitics and disciplinary development of engineering education: A case study. *Discourse: Studies in the cultural politics of education, 35*(2), 266–277.

Bowen, G. A. (2010). From qualitative dissertation to quality articles: Seven lessons learned. *Qualitative Report, 15*(4), 864–879.

Caputo, J., & Yount, M. (Eds.) (1993). *Foucault and the critique of institutions.* University Park: Pennsylvania State University Press.

Crescentini, A., & Mainardi, G. (2009). Qualitative research articles: guidelines, suggestions and needs. *Journal of Workplace Learning, 21*(5), 431–439.

Duran, R. P., Eisenhart, M. A., Erickson, F. D., Grant, C. A., Green, J. L., Hedges, L. V., Levine, F. J., et al. (2006). Standards for reporting on empirical social science research in AERA Publications American Educational Research Association. *Educational Researcher, 35*(6), 33–40.

Elsevier. (n.d.). Retrieved April 27, 2012, from www.elsevier.com/wps/find/reviewershome.reviewers/reviewersguidelines

Flynn, T. (2005). Foucault's mapping of history. In G. Gutting (Ed.), *The Cambridge companion to Foucault* (second edition) (pp. 29–48). Cambridge, UK: Cambridge University Press.

Foucault, M. (1972). *The archaeology of knowledge and the discourse on language.* A. M. Sheridan Smith (Trans.). New York: Pantheon Books.

Foucault, M. (1978). *The history of sexuality: an introduction* (volume 1). New York: Vintage.

Foucault, M. (1980). *Power/Knowledge: Selected interviews and other writings, 1972–1977.* C. Cordon, L. Marshall, J. Mepham, & K. Soper(Trans.). C. Cordon (Ed.). New York: Pantheon Books.

Foucault, M. (1983). Afterword: the subject and power. In H. Dreyfus & P. Rabinow (Eds.), *Michel Foucault: beyond structuralism and hermeneutics* (second edition) (pp. 208–226). Chicago: University of Chicago Press.

Foucault, M. (1984). Polemics, politics, and problematizations. In P. Rabinow (Ed.), *The Foucault reader* (pp. 381–390). New York: Pantheon.

Foucault, M. (2003). *"Society must be defended." Lectures at the College de France (1975–76).* D. Macey (Trans.).). New York: Picador.

Foucault, M., Burchell, G., Gordon, C., & Miller, P. (1991). *The Foucault effect: Studies in governmentality : With two lectures by and an interview with Michel Foucault.* Chicago: University of Chicago Press.

Frank, J. (2013). Mitigating against epistemic injustice in educational research. *Educational Researcher, 42*(7), 363–370.

Greckhamer, T., Koro-Ljungberg, M., Cilesiz, S., & Hayes, S. (2008). Demystifying interdisciplinary qualitative research. *Qualitative Inquiry, 14*(2), 307–331.

Kasman, D. L. (2003). Knowledge as power: The impact of normativity on epistemology. *The American Journal of Bioethics, 3*(2), 20–22.

Kendall, G., & Wickham, G. (2000). *Using Foucault's methods.* London and Thousand Oaks, CA: Sage.

Koro-Ljungberg, M. (2010). Validity, responsibility, and aporia. *Qualitative Inquiry, 16* (8), 603–610.

Koro-Ljungberg, M., Carlson, D., Tesar, M., & Anderson, K. (in press). Methodology *brut*: Philosophy, ecstatic thinking, and some other (unfinished) things. *Qualitative Inquiry.*

Kotowski, M. R., & Miller, L. E. (2010). The mpact of interdisciplinary collaboration. *Health Communication, 25*(6/7), 567–568.

Langfeldt, L. (2006). The policy challenges of peer review: Managing bias, conflict of interests and interdisciplinary assessments. *Research Evaluation, 15*(1), 31–41.

Lather, P. (1994). Fertile obsession: Validity after poststructuralism. In A. D. Gitlin (Ed.), *Power and method: Political activism and educational research* (pp. xii, 248 p.). New York: Routledge.

Laudel, G. (2006). Conclave in the Tower of Babel: How peers review interdisciplinary research proposals. *Research Evaluation, 15*(1), 57–68.

Lorenzetti, D. L., & Rutherford, G. (2012). Information professionals' participation in interdisciplinary research: A preliminary study of factors affecting successful collaborations. *Health Information & Libraries Journal, 29*(4), 274–284.

Maxwell, J. (2010). Validity: How might you be wrong? In W. Luttrell (Ed.), *Qualitative educational research: Readings in reflexive methodology and transformative practice* (pp. 279–287). New York: Routledge.

Scheurich, J. J. (1996). The masks of validity: A deconstructive investigation. *International Journal of Qualitative Studies in Education, 9*(1), 49–60.

Schoenberg, N. E., & McAuley, W. J. (2007). Promoting qualitative research. *The Gerontologist, 47*(5), 576–577.

Taylor, E. W., Beck, J., & Ainsworth, E. (2001). Publishing qualitative adult education research: A peer review perspective. *Studies in the Education of Adults, 33*(2), 163–179.

Wolcott, H. (1990). On seeking—and rejecting—validity in qualitative research. In E. Eisner & A. Peshkin (Eds.), *Qualitative inquiry in education: Continuing the debate* (pp. 121–152). New York: Teachers College, Columbia University.

Zaruba, K. E., Toma, J. D., & Stark, J. S. (1996). Criteria used for qualitative research in the refereeing process. *Review of Higher Education, 19*(4), 435–460.

Chapter 2

Critical Qualitative Research in Global Neoliberalism

Foucault, Inquiry, and Transformative Possibilities

Gaile S. Cannella and Yvonna S. Lincoln

Descriptions and critiques of our contemporary hyper-capitalist condition abound, from the range of critical, poststructural, feminist, anti-colonial perspectives, to even economic analysis. Capitalist power networks have been, to some extent, exposed in the marginalized locations of academia. Some scholars even refer to the condition as the most recent version of patriarchy, as capitalist patriarchy (Eisenstein, 1999; von Werlhof, 2007). Yet, this "canon of critique" (Kincheloe, 2008, p. 14) has not resulted in societal transformation. This lack of transformation toward social justice has been, most often, attributed to the increasing globalization of Western neoliberal ways of being, power networks associated with capitalism, the privileging of free market ideologies, profiteering, and managerial orientations. Although, from various academic perspectives over the past 50 years, calls for a critical social science have been articulated and concerns regarding capitalism have been foundational to economic anxieties within those appeals, capitalism has spread rhizomatically through previously uninvaded spaces. We are concerned that thought/action/language/being are increasingly difficult unless using a neoliberal 'voice,' and impossible without at

Qualitative Inquiry and the Politics of Research edited by Norman K. Denzin and Michael D. Giardina, 51–74. © 2015 Left Coast Press, Inc. All rights reserved.

least a neoliberal 'accent.' This contemporary global neoliberal context demands an immediate infusion, and movement to the center, of a critical social science that radically researches power and possibilities for resistance(s) and generates critical counter actions on the ground.

For some time now, various scholars, individuals, and groups have called for, and used traditionally marginalized perspectives to construct, critical research conceptualizations and practices. As an example, Pinar (2001) illustrates this type of inquiry in an extensive, in-depth (1,200 page history) study of racial violence in the United States from the antebellum and post-Reconstruction South to post-1960s prisons, using lynching and prison rape as the focus. Pinar juxtaposes viewpoints from traditionally marginalized scholars who would queer the gaze of historical research analysis (a practice that some recently refer to as thinking with theory). Further, he acknowledges his intimate connection with those perspectives. He demonstrates interrelatedness between sex, gender, and race, making "visible a mangled and repressed homoeroticism lacing white men's hatred of black" to violent acts (p. 3). Creating research that emanates from the range of radical critical positions has also been described as a "third moment" of qualitative inquiry (Denzin & Giardina, 2009, p. 21). Further, other examples employ viewpoints like Black feminist thought, Chicana feminisms, and the range of Indigenous knowledges (Cannella & Manuelito, 2008; Collins, 2000; Smith, 1999; Trujillo, 1998), as well as the range of critical and feminist scholarly perspectives.

In his 1970s lectures, Foucault referred to critical work as "the insurrection of subjugated knowledges" or "returns of knowledge" (1997, English translation, 2003, p. 7). He included both buried and masked historical contents and the range of knowledges that have traditionally been disqualified as non-conceptual, illogical, or otherwise placed in the margins and made invisible. We would also include the perspectives of scholars who, although sometimes even white and educationally privileged, have been placed in the margins of Western, male, white, and rationalist research hegemony. Please note that we avoid using terms like *theory* as much as possible, and potentially even conceptualizations like thinking, because of ties (although often hidden) to dominant, dualistic, even deterministic discourses. These diverse perspectives can/do, however, serve as multi-foundational to constructions of critical social science—as vantage points—as organizational structures—as emergent challenges to research from within the process—as positions that generate multiple and diverse contingencies. Quoting Kincheloe, "Simply in the act of attending to and learning from the insights of marginalized peoples, we operate as allies in their struggle" (2008, p. 6).

From within this contemporary location of critical possibility, the purpose of this chapter is to employ a critical stance that has been predominantly either dismissed or obscured as related to the neoliberal condition. The perspectives with which we plan to interact are those expressed in Foucault's discussions of neoliberalism in *Society Must be Defended* (2003) and *The Birth of Biopolitics* (2008), as well as scholarly reactions to those lectures. Although we understand that the histories generated by Foucault are not at all marginalized in our critical sphere, the research is either ostracized or used to reinscribe oppressive past presents in academia more broadly. Additionally, we do share the belief that the use of the work of white, male scholars is always/already problematic in our struggle to center marginalized perspectives, even if these scholars are critical. However, and acknowledging the somewhat related work of Lemke (2011) and Rose (1999), we feel that Foucaultian genealogies of neoliberalisms are not widely considered in the construction of critical research that would challenge neoliberalism. Therefore, we choose to make use of our readings of Foucault's discussions of neoliberalisms and Homo economicus as the point from which to generate critical research questions. Further, because most of us have direct, on the ground, personal experiences with higher education (even if not our chosen field of study) and our homes in higher education should certainly be locations for critical action (if that action is possible anywhere), the current neoliberal infusion in higher education around the globe serves as our example.

Transformed Liberal Doctrines: Invasive Neoliberal Saturations

In the *Birth of Biopolitics* (2008), genealogies of two centuries of liberalism, and *Society Must Be Defended* (2003), Foucault problematizes the two major neoliberal schools, German ordoliberalism and American anarcho-liberalism. Additionally, references to French constructions, especially after the revolution, and British political radicalism are employed. Although the discourses are not considered an exact match, there are major neoliberal commonalities and certainly overlaps and interactions, as global travels and technologies have blurred the boundaries.

As we share our deep reading of these neoliberal genealogies, we set the stage by offering an overly simplistic description of the notion of liberalism, not as a truth oriented definition of a complex and multiple ideology, but as a reference point for our conversation and research constructions. Liberalism can be considered an ideology committed to limited government (avoiding sovereign powers) and individual rights (individual liberties that also include the free market). Most associate liberalism with capitalism, which is a complexity that will not be directly addressed or defined in this chapter. However, this complexity (and the need for the inclusion of capitalism) cannot be avoided when one considers that liberal ideologies split into groups: classical liberals who believe in small government but support industry, and social liberals who believe in government intervention that would support equity and protection for all citizens. Broadly, according to Foucault (2008), liberal perspectives have historically privileged market economy, but have defined that privilege as exchange, an exchange that engages partners who must be protected through oversight and regulation (the consumer being one of those partners). In his problematization of the neoliberal condition, Foucault proposes major shifts literally in all ways/aspects of living and being (a biopolitics) away from the focus on markets, exchange, and oversight that have dominated the two hundred year history of liberalism. Rather, neoliberalism has become a form of embodiment that no longer functions to protect the various partners engaged through exchange; neoliberalism is a present, multiple, and becoming assemblage that encompasses all aspects of being (whether thought or unthought) for the purposes of competition, enterprise, and the reinvigoration and reterritorialization of itself (Delueze & Guatarri, 1977, 1987).

Although clearly different in a range of ways, neoliberal practices in the United States and various European countries all developed within contexts that were, to some extent, reactionary to more classical liberal forms of governmentality. In the United States, as examples, the New Deal, guaranteed jobs for soldiers following WWII, and federal growth through social programs in the Johnson administration are discussed by Foucault (and others) as conditions from which emerged neoliberal critique and counter discourses. Additionally, different liberal histories have undergone continual internal debate, creating broad-based conditions for territorializations by neoliberal perspectives. American liberalism has a "foothold in both the right and the left. It is also a sort of utopian focus which is always being revived. It is also a method of thought, a grid of economic and sociological analysis" (Foucault, 2008, p. 218). Complicated by the right's privileging of liberalism's rejection of anything interpreted as socialist and the left's avoidance of the construction of a military state, forms of liberalism have dominated political debate in the United States throughout its history. Issues of nation, independence, or the Rule of Law have been more likely recurrent elements in Europe (Foucault, 2008), and the liberal debate has been less inclusive, but influential. To illustrate, the post French Revolution method of setting juridical limits to the power of public authority, called "Rousseau's approach" (p. 39), attempted to define individual, natural, even original rights, as well as the condition under which the exchange or ceding of those rights was accepted. Further, perspectives like English political radicalism attempted to determine what government would be useful to do, to verify both pointless and beneficial forms of interference. Diverse (and conflicting) conceptualizations of the law and of freedom characterize the ambiguity in European liberalism. However, as transformations from liberalism to neoliberalism have progressed, governmentality broadly, and in diverse locations, has certainly become a major issue.

Probably the most common concern invoked by those fearful of our current neoliberal condition, is market privilege, rampant consumerism/materialism, and, of course, hyper/super capitalism. However, Foucault proposes that neoliberalism represents a major shift more broadly, a transformation that goes outside and beyond ideology, but is rather a complete saturation. "Neoliberalism is not Adam Smith; neoliberalism is not market society; neoliberalism is not the Gulag on the insidious scale of capitalism" (Foucault, 2008, p. 131). In neoliberalism, the market has shifted from the liberal site of exchange and regulation for justice and jurisdiction to a site of veridiction, the location, generator, embodiment of the rules of verification and falsification. Market economy as represented by a massive privileging of competition has become the determiner of the rules for what can be said/not said, accepted as truth/disqualified, performed or acted upon/rejected. Neoliberalism "is the idea that the economy is basically a game, that is developed as a game, ... that the whole of society must be permeated by this economic game, and that the essential role of the state is to define the economic rules of the game" (p. 201). Principles of a market economy are to be the standards for the exercise of political power.

At this point in our discussion of Foucault's perspectives (and to assist us with space and clarity), we want to discuss three major themes that are helpful as we struggle to construct new research purposes within an increasingly global neoliberal condition. These themes are (1) the neoliberal reconstruction/privileging/protection of an economics of competition, (2) Homo entrepreneur, the individual, human body of enterprise, and (3) saturation so complete that ideology is not necessary and is made invisible.

Privileging/Protecting an Economics of Competition

As mentioned previously, the market focus in neoliberalism is competition rather than exchange. Privileging *competition* denounces practices of laissez-faire government. In neoliberalism, all possibilities for competition must be facilitated and protected, therefore requiring government intervention. Yet, this economics of competition is not about equal access or fairness, but rather privatization, enterprise, and capital. Further, human nature is constructed as competitive; 'competitive nature' must be guarded/ assisted/facilitated. But, this protection is to safeguard the economics of competition, not human nature. The purpose of government is to secure "the social and legal framework necessary to promote unfettered competition" (Sawicki, 2013).

The question is not: Into what should we intervene? Facilitating an economics of competition is believed to require intervention into all aspects of society, although not necessarily obviously or always directly. The question is: Just how should something be touched; what is the style of governance? "Legal, geographic, scientific, social factors become objects of government intervention that would follow the market framework policy. How can we modify these things so the market economy can come into play?" (Foucault, 2008, p. 141). Regulatory and organizing structures are considered entirely appropriate if facilitating competition.

The neoliberal focus on competition also turns upside down constructs and protections that have commonly been associated with liberal governmentality. We have already mentioned the reconceptualization of the system of jurisdiction to veridiction. Constructs like 'monopoly' are also considered false issues, with a range of neoliberal scholars putting forward theories as to how/why such concerns are unnecessary. In addition to examining/ unmasking these neoliberal conceptualizations, Foucault summarizes the view: "Monopolistic phenomenon does not belong in principle or logically to the economics of competition" (p. 135). "There is no need to intervene directly in the economic process, since the economic process, as the bearer itself of a regulatory structure in the form of competition, will never go wrong if it is allowed to function fully" (p. 137). For an economics of competition, there is no fear of, or concern about, monopoly. This logic may appear contradictory, but it simply stated (although not simply applied) is used to eliminate protections for the various partners in exchange while increasing forms of governmentality (and literally government performed interventions) that create new privileges for competitive economics (e.g., privatizing traditional public services, constructing practices that define individual human beings in relation to forms of measurement and capital, rather than as always valued affirmations of life, nature, and complex connections).

In an enterprise society constructed by neoliberalism and now subject to the dynamics of unfettered competition, conceptualizations of social policy are also reformulated. Rather than social policy to insure the welfare of citizens, social policy is defined as economic growth and privatization. The economic game is believed to be the societal regulator; therefore inequality must be allowed to exist:

> Government must not form a counterpoint or a screen, as it were, between society and economic processes. It has to intervene on society as such, in its fabric and depth. Basically, it has to intervene on society so that competitive mechanisms can play a regulatory role at every moment and every point in society, and by intervening in this way its objective will become possible, that is to say, a general regulation of society by the market. (Foucault, 2008, p. 145)

Entrepreneurialism: Self as Human Capital

Within neoliberalism, a technology of the self is constructed. This technology involves a shift in human subjectivity toward human nature as competitive. Again, this nature must be protected— not the individual, rather the competitive nature. The old label, *Homo economicus,* is used—but, rather than man of exchange, or consumer—neoliberal homo economicus is "man of enterprise and production" (Foucault, 2008, p. 147). This man of production is now *Homo entrepreneur.* "In practice, the stake in all neo-liberal analysis is … homo economicus as entrepreneur of himself, being for himself his own capital, being for himself his own producer, being for himself the source of (his) earnings" (p. 226).

Homo entrepreneur is now the capital, literally the human capital, the physical body of income. Entrepreneurial functioning and development of the skills and achievements toward that functioning are the ways of living and being. Human beings, most in the past referred to as workers, are no longer oppositional to their capitalist bosses. Rather, each human being is to view her/himself as an economic and broad-based corporation of one, the body responsible for all choices. The individual now embodies the income, and functions with a self-interested governmentality, an egocentric body of innovation, enterprise, and productivity. All human actions are viewed as investments and the responsibility of the individual.

Human capital is made up of two components. The first is heredity, the extent to which the individual is born as a naturally competitive, innovative, entrepreneurial body. This notion obviously provokes anxiety in those who would challenge neoliberalism as racism and sexism and so forth can be legitimated within the human capital discourse, but also as a perspective that places all responsibility upon the human body. The second component is the environment, or more appropriately, what the human individual does to improve him/herself as a capital being in the environment. This improvement includes that which is acquired though education, cultural stimuli, or other forms of intervention. This individual investment in human capital is what is considered to account for economic gain (and 'success' in all aspects of life). As an example, when Foucault conducted the 1970s lectures, he described how financial problems in so-called Third World economies are interpreted by neoliberalism as lack of investment in human capital rather than colonial past presents, historical pilfering of resources from outside powers, and/ or blockage in economic mechanisms by those with privilege.

This focus on human capital has become a regime of veridiction that legitimates two processes: (1) infusion of economic interpretations into previously uninvaded territories or domains, and therefore, (2) construction of the non-economic as economic (and so tied to capital). These processes then serve to create the conditions for saturation (a situation that will be discussed next).

Finally, Homo entrepreneur as a broad-based model for human subjectivity has become the norm, a specter or ghostly presence in all human endeavor (Marttila, 2013). This version of "homo economicus is someone who is eminently governable" (Foucault, 2008, p. 270). The entrepreneur is a person who accepts neoliberal reality and dutifully and rationally attempts to modify environmental variables as needed. As examples, Foucault refers to sets of techniques used in the United States, like behavior modification and practices in the field of psychiatry that easily engage with economic analysis, notions of human capital, and the entrepreneurial body as producer and income. Neoliberal Homo entrepreneur is precisely the body built to be managed.

Neoliberal Saturations: Capitalism without Capitalism and/or Neoliberalism without Neoliberalism

Neoliberalism is not an ideology, but a total emersion within competition and enterprise formation throughout daily life, politics, government, and action. Some have referred to this as capitalism without capitalism, or neoliberalism without neoliberalism. The infiltration is so complete that the condition is made invisible—*saturation* without the requirement of ideological examination or acceptance. Alternatives are viewed as impossible within this environment of intensification.

Rather than directly marking bodies, knowledge, actions, or even the environment neoliberal forms of governmentality surreptitiously penetrate, invade, and construct all human behavior, including the invasion of bodies. Marketing principles of management are facilitated by the state and defined through cost benefit analysis. Neoliberalism applies economic analysis to all forms of behavior, domains of conduct, forms of knowledge—whether marriage, education, or constructions of criminality—silently invading perspectives, even ideologies like religion, historical fields, and definitely the individual.

Challenging/Resisting Neoliberalism

On the cover of *Society Must be Defended* (2003) is written, "Above all, Foucault shows, power is not an external force, but a subtle form of control that we all consent to uphold." Many have decried the work of Foucault as depressing and as if eliminating possibilities for human agency, and after being exposed to his discussions of neoliberalism, some might agree with this assessment. However, others suggest just the opposite (Butin, 2001; Sawicki, 2013; Winnubst, 2012), and we agree. His very conceptualizations of power as nonexistent without resistance, as exercised/infused rather than hierarchal, provide prospects for critical actions that would counter and even deterritorialize neoliberalism (Thompson, 2003).

Additionally, Foucault ultimately discusses the ways that liberalism has continued to critique and debate governmental practice in Europe and how Americans have continuously been haunted by the anxieties, demands, and questions of liberalism. "It is the object of public debate regarding its 'good or bad,' its 'too much or too little'" (Foucault, 2008, p. 322). Various ways of examining conditions that support particular regimes of veridiction are being explored through critical qualitative research. These understandings, the power and ambiguities of societies and individuals, and the complexities of power/resistance can facilitate all manner of action and transformation.

Foucault further proposes genealogies of regimes of veridiction that include both rule and transformations of rule by truth saturations. "All these cases—whether it is the market, the confessional, the psychiatric institution, or the prison—involve taking up a history of truth under different angles, or rather, taking up a history of truth that is coupled, from the start, with a history of law" (2008, p. 35). Researching neoliberalism must include the recognition of the doubled jurisdictional function transformed (and multiplied) by addition of neoliberal veridiction. The cause cannot be found and should not be pursued, and so (according to Foucault) will not be the purpose of research. Rather, establishing the "intelligibility of the process by describing the connection between different phenomena" (p. 33) is necessary. Additionally, the connections, processes, and the rules of veridiction cannot be considered deductive. Research, and forms of activism concerned with the damages of neoliberalism, can employ a recognition of the schizophrenic invasion of capitalism described by Deleuze and Guatarri (1977, 1987) as rhyzomatic, flexible and reterritorializing, and even becoming (Foucault, 1977) to generate an always/already awareness of the complexities of the current condition. Finally, diverse ways of living and traditionally marginalized perspectives can, if placed in the center, generate a range of possibilities (Cannella, 2014; Cannella, Perez & Pasque, 2015; Eisenstein, 1999; Klein, 2014).

Foucault, Activism, and Reconceptualizing Research

Since Foucault's genealogical work has been overly critiqued, especially in the field of education, as constructing the human subject as lacking agency, and therefore dismal, depressing, and ultimately lacking in societal options, the fallacies of this perspective must be briefly addressed in any discussion related to Foucault's interpretations of neoliberalism. Interpretations of the scholarship as constructing perspectives in which human beings lack agency, in which resistance is excluded, or that are relativistic, ignore major positions found in the work as well as Foucault's own history of activism (Felski, 1998; Macey, 1993). "Today, new fools, or the same ones reincarnated [*in reference to people who were surprised at Spinoza's wish for the liberation of man centuries ago; explanation added by this author*] are astonished because Foucault, who had spoken of the death of man, took part in political struggle" (Delueze, 1988).

Butin (2001) discusses the ways that the very foundation of Foucault's work represents possibilities for a liberatory and activist stance. Underlying pessimistic interpretations of the work is a constrained, limited understanding of power—as if power is a limited, disciplinary, unidirectional relation. For Foucault, however, power relations are never simply good/bad, active/reactive, dominant/oppressive, but can always be dangerous and therefore require continued critique. More importantly, power relations do not exist without agency from multiple points and multiple actors; Foucault's notion of power relations would collapse without agents capable of acting (Butin, 2001). "These power relations are thus mobile, reversible, and unstable" (Foucault, 1997, p. 292). Further, power itself is viewed as necessarily embodying resistance. "In power relations there is necessarily the possibility of resistance because if there were no possibility of resistance (of violent resistance, flight, deception, strategies capable of reversing the situation), there would be no power relations at all" (Foucault, 1997, p. 292). For this conceptualization of power relations, possibilities for resistance are always present (even to the point of choosing to die), whether one chooses to resist or not.

If there are relations of power in every social field, this is because there is freedom everywhere. Of course, states of domination do indeed exist. In a great many cases, power relations are fixed in such a way that they are perpetually asymmetrical and allow an extremely limited margin of freedom.... In such cases of domination, be they economic, social, institutional, or sexual, the problem is knowing where resistance will (can) develop. (Foucault, 1997, p. 291)

Reconceptualizing Research

Regarding inquiry (and also notions of relativism), Foucault describes his position as not apathetic, but as a kind of hyper-activism. Vigilant critique and resistance involves daily examination of power relations. "I think that the ethico-political choice we have to make every day is to determine which is the main danger" (Foucault, 1997, p. 256). Further, solutions to problems are not viewed as grounded in past solutions (whether research or forms of activism), or in determining new truths. Rather, solutions are grounded in the genealogies of new problems, in the history of the construction of power relations related to the particular problem, and especially by demonstrating that there are other reasonable options. "One escapes from a domination of truth not by playing a game that [is] totally different from the game of truth, but by playing the same game differently, or playing another game ... with other trump cards" (Foucault, 1997, p. 295).

This Foucaultian research perspective avoids taking a normalizing stance or a disposition that would provide definitive answers or ask "why?" Truth oriented answers are expected when "why?" is the question; examining "how" regulatory practices function generates possibilities for both exposure and experimentation with new ways of being (Butin, 2001). Further, the broader disposition is to map strategic games so that different rules, moves, and uses for resources can be constructed (Sawacki, 2013), and to empirically acknowledge examples of resistance and struggle (Butin, 2001).

The focus of a critical qualitative research could ultimately become "linking together as tightly as possible the historical and theoretical analysis of power relations, institutions, and knowledge, to the movements, critiques, and experiences that call them into question in reality" (Foucault, 1984, p. 374). More specifically, in order to understand power relations, and increase possibilities for transformation, inquiry is necessary into "forms of resistance and attempts made to dissociate these relations" (Foucault, 1982, p. 211), new/unthought options for transforming power relations, and engagement with resistance and struggle.

Research and Activism in Neoliberalism

While avoiding normalizing perspectives and practices, Foucault's research purposes are to provide possibilities for "playing the game differently." Although some of us (ourselves included) are very uncomfortable with referring to the power relations that impact our very existence as a "game," perhaps the use of this term periodically in relation to neoliberalism is a more optimistic position. Illustrative strategies include, but are not limited to, the focus on resistance and on using, and potentially constructing, existing societal (and individual) resources differently.

The first illustration is to focus on Foucault's agenda regarding resistance. As mentioned previously, resistance is inherent in relations of power from a Foucaultian perspective; further, power cannot exist without resistance (and agency) from all locations (even those of the most marginalized and oppressed). Foucault's project was/is to reveal openings for resistance, understandings of options. The purpose is not to assure or even promote resistance, but rather to concede opportunities (Butin, 2001). From this perspective, power is always considered complex and intersecting, and agency (in some form) is always possible. Research can inquire into: forms of resistance applied by the many who live within difficult power relations all around us; how particular forms of resistance support particular perspectives and new ways of playing the game; and what a willingness to resist tells us about those who would struggle. Understanding the multiple practices of, and decisions about, resistance generates and allows for entirely different perspectives on power relations. Sedgwick (2003) challenges us to look for the ways that those who live with intolerable and oppressive conditions find pleasure and humor, the "middle ranges of agency" (p. 13), that may create new spaces for change.

A second illustration is Foucault's focus on the use of cultural resources differently. While the ultimate use of the master's tools can always be questioned (Lorde, 1984), turning those tools upside down to generate counter forces, or new territories, is also possible. One complex example is Foucault's notion of self-constitution and ethics (Sawicki, 2013). Some scholars have critiqued his notion of the individual as consistent with the neoliberal imposition of the self as enterprise (McNay, 2009; Oksala, 2005). Others believe that, from within neoliberalism and to potentially escape or transform its power relations, a reconstituting of self (a working on the self) in ways that experiment with "forming other ways of life, new forms of rationality, understandings of self, and habits of relating to oneself and others" (Sawicki, 2013, p. 84) is necessary as a critical practice personally and professionally. This perspective can turn upside down and inside out the liberal and neoliberal economic, capitalist, and rationalist notions of the individual (Dilts, 2010). Sawicki (2013) points out that Foucault aimed to "show us that we are 'freer than we feel,' that in actuality we are not always trapped within the trends that we capture in our reflections upon what is happening in the present" (Foucault, 1988, p. 10; in Sawicki, 2013, p. 84). This very perspective would suggest that our research, and our practices as researchers, can focus on "cultivating other forms of life, other types of relational possibilities and understandings," and on "keeping possibilities for non-entrepreneurial self-relationships alive" (p. 85). This reconstitution of an ethical self, that is no longer predominantly competitive, entrepreneurial, or economic, can literally become a site for the critical reconceptualization of research purposes and practices. From within this reading of Foucaultian genealogies of neoliberalism and purposes for critical research practices/actions, we now move to considerations within contemporary neoliberal transformations in higher education.

Reconceptualizing Research in the Condition of Neoliberal Higher Education

Globally, a range of scholars have expressed concern regarding the shifts in higher education toward neoliberalism, even as far as inquiry into the construction of the corporate, military, university, industrial complex (Cannella & Miller, 2008). This work is absolutely needed and has revealed the changes in funding, administration and governance, as well as the redistribution of resources and changes in academic workers (Amit, 2000; Lincoln, 2011, 2012a, 2012b; Slaughter & Rhoades, 2004). This scholarship should continue and be made more public by expanding methods of dissemination. Additionally, the field of qualitative research is ideal as a location for critical work that challenges neoliberalism in higher education in a variety of ways (Cannella, 2014). Specifically, the field has been well developed in a broad range of academic areas that include, but are not limited to, education, sociology and justice studies, communication studies, and medicine. Additionally, qualitative data construction and collection practices like interviewing, participant observation, document and image analyses, and journaling, as well as broad ranging forms of discourse analyses (that are not simple language analytic forms), are ideal for critical purposes when partnered with diverse, traditionally marginalized perspectives. Finally, critical scholarship from diverse perspectives, like feminisms, queer theory, and anti-colonialism, provides a wealth of models. This work can all be used to construct a body of critical scholarship and critical action specific to the local and global neoliberal conditions of/in higher education. However, related specifically to Foucault's discussions of neoliberalism, we want to suggest the range of research possibilities that can by their own practices and existence serve as counter discourses, and hopefully counter actions. We make these suggestions using the themes incorporated into our previous discussions: economics of competition, notions of human capital, and neoliberalism that saturates all aspects of life and being.

Economics of Competition

Higher education has become the object, producer, and embodiment of neoliberalism and the economics of competition through intervention, construction of competitive organizing structures and competitive truth as regulator, the transformation of higher education social policy into support for growth and privatization, and a construction, and privileging, of inequality. An environment that is grounded in competition and capitalism's need for growth has emerged as higher education as a major site for information and knowledge production has been invaded and coopted. Ranking systems (Lincoln, 2012b) are used to literally intervene into all fields, forms of knowledge, and practices of inquiry as journals, faculty, programs, and institutions themselves are placed under ordered (and simplistic) surveillance, categorized, and labeled. Further, these systems are used to create hierarchical competitive organizing structures that produce inequality through the construction of scientific priesthoods and funded idols who do not question neoliberalism or privileged forms of research; much of the work is used to further privatize that which has always been public. The competitive structure is perpetuated and rewarded; bodies that challenge or question that structure are placed in the margins, and even erased (e.g., 'disestablishment' of colleges, programs, fields at particular institutions).

As critical qualitative researchers, our focus can be to unveil current practices and generate new opportunities for sites of resistance that are not competitive. This research can/should include continued practices of genealogy and deconstruction, but also new purposes and methodologies that involve direct action and understandings of practices of resistance. Broad-based areas of emphasis can include (but are not limited to):

> Continued inquiry into systems of power relations (e.g., historically how neoliberalism has invaded, and reconstituted as competitive, particular conceptualizations/aspects/practices of higher education; "deep critical examination of the subterranean changes in our institutions" (Lincoln, 2012a, p. 3), such as changes in promotion and tenure over time);

> Research into activism and public forms of dissemination related to these power relations;

> Inquiry into forms and practices of resistance currently performed in neoliberal higher education (e.g., forms of publication resistance as described by Goetsch, 2010) along with ways to make public across academia these new options for resistance;

Recognition of the continued struggle for transformation by experimenting with forms of domination (power relations) that may be less dangerous (e.g., employing subjugated knowledges, placing economic/capitalism in the margin); and

Academic collaborations that think research, academic practices, and higher education organizations and administration differently with expectations for scholarly work that is ethical, reparative, and useful for always/already addressing power relations, but that is not competitive (or at least counters competition at multiple points).

Entrepreneurialism: Self as Human Capital

The notion of human capital within higher education creates faculty as literally the self-interested, physical body of income as played out in the focus on grant writing, publication counts, patents, and reinscriptions of quantitative accountability constructs like mixed methods research, evidenced-based practices, and large data bases. Individual human beings were already expected to be productive and, to some extent, entrepreneurial in the practice of higher education. However, this expectation is taken farther as everyone is to be enterprising and innovative, not 'simply' concerned with and even passionate about societal and/or environmental issues—now this passion must lead to funding, patents for the university, and increased capital. The attracting of external funds, ties to private industry, and deterministic answers to problems are now the major focus as entrepreneurialism is now the specter for all human endeavor.

The attempt in Texas to require faculty to generate their own salaries by creating profit-loss reports for faculty is an example conceptually. The report constructs implications about who is worth his or her income by exploring who generates capital from outside (Lincoln, 2010), also resulting in a discourse that would eliminate state responsibility for the common good (further reinscribing the neoliberal saturation more broadly). Individuals are ultimately judged, disqualified, and/or literally rewarded from this neoliberal, objective distance. "Those whom we deem most valuable as an information-economy object, institutions will seek to keep, and those least valuable in the same terms institutions will permit to leave readily" (Lincoln, 2012b, p. 457).

The individual (in this case the faculty member, graduate student, or administrator) is held responsible for his or her own intellect and environmental interventions (like education, or training, or practicing research in a particular manner) that facilitate survival in the neoliberal academy. Further, dutifully functioning within that climate as the academic entrepreneur is considered absolutely necessary for promotion, tenure, and other recognitions and rewards. As mentioned previously, Foucault describes this entrepreneurial, productive, innovative physical body as the ultimate being made to be governed—managed without whip or lash—by neoliberal expectations that would have her or him live/function/be as capital.

This notion of the academic entrepreneur can be interpreted as a power relation that cannot be resisted. However, both practices of resistance and reconstitutions of the ethical self afford opportunities to counter the human capital construct in higher education. Example broad-based research and action possibilities include:

> Inquire into historical case studies of the construction of faculty and/or student subjectivities (e.g., employment expectations; involvement in governance);
>
> Work collaboratively to construct "justice" subjectivities (individually and as research groups)—becomings that are aware of what's happening to all in the community;
>
> Reconceptualize dominant research tools in practice (which has been done in qualitative research though construction of a range of methodologies, publication outlets, conferences, etc.) that can challenge neoliberalism;
>
> As one engages with reconstitution of self as researcher, conduct research continuously addressing issues like: ethical substance, mode of subjectification, ethical work, and telos:
>
>> How do we avoid political technologies of the individual and continue to be researchers who must often perform as individuals?

> What new modes of ethical relations do I invent within the practices of my research? (See Cannella, 2014; Cannella & Lincoln, 2011; Lincoln & Cannella, 2007)

Construct researcher self as activist, acknowledging that "if we don't provide the counter narratives, who will?" (Lincoln, 2012a, p. 11).

Our responsibility to the public and to ourselves is to generate possibilities. Academic scholarship and researchers should never be limited by a dominant way of being. Foucault discusses the idea that his work is to create options for resistance not necessarily to promote resistance. However, we do believe that our responsibility is to resist saturations that limit—remembering that as researchers we are privileged—our purpose is not to be managed, but rather to ethically expand possibilities—to continuously critique power relations and take actions based on agendas that would (as needed) attempt transformations. These actions may be dangerous for our professional lives, and will usually 'brand' us as trouble makers, not smart enough to obtain grants, or any number of other derogatory labels. However, as researchers and scholars, can we expect anyone else to challenge neoliberalism if we are not willing to do so?

Neoliberal Saturations

Many are rightfully concerned that neoliberal successes may have embedded us within "a malaise from which higher education may not recover" (Lincoln, 2012a, p. 2). Although throughout this chapter we have used Foucault's perspectives to demand that resistance is always possible, we understand that transforming this new form of saturation that has both invaded all aspects of our lives and gone beyond the most complex of ideologies may be considered impossible. However, as already demonstrated, revealing forms of resistance that exist in higher education as well as diverse locations all around us, and transforming dominant cultural resources (even constructions of ourselves as individuals) to challenge, rethink, and perhaps move toward more equitable power relations is always possible. "In power relations, there is necessarily the possibility of resistance" (Foucault, 1997, p. 292). As researchers, we must:

Experiment with forms of counter conduct within higher education, researching and disseminating the new practices (e.g., direct counter actions on the ground that involve the public in communication and practice, conceptualzing a culture that is supportive and avoids control, countering audit culture from within);

Research the unthought regarding knowledge and ways of being by constructing agendas that do not privilege economics in any form (e.g., generating ways to place justice at the forefront in higher education; constructing new forms of faculty support; creating unthought sites for critical information commons);

Construct and research broad-based locations for academic work and scholarship, locations that may create new partnerships, but that always/already avoid practices that facilitate private enterprise or capitalist productions; and

Research ways to collaborate and work together that are not competitive or entrepreneurial, but that place at the forefront a notion of the common good that develops a considerate and concerned community, facilitates possibilities for both social and environmental justice, and creates higher education as a location that facilitates welfare and unlimited possibilities.

We certainly live within an increasingly global, invasive, and rhizomatic neoliberalism. Yet, all power relations, even those produced within and producing neoliberalism, are flexible, changing, embedded within resistance, and can be transformed. As scholars and researchers, we must optimistically believe that transformation is possible. We must, however, also be willing to spend the time and take the risks necessary to reveal, generate, and act on these possibilities.

References

Amit, V. (2000). The university as panopticon: Moral claims and attacks on academic freedom. In M. Strathern (Ed.), *Audit cultures* (pp. 215–234). New York: Routledge.

Butin, S. W. (2001). If this is resistance I would hate to see domination: Retrieving Foucault's notion of resistance within educational research. *Educational Studies, 32* (2), 157–176.

Cannella, G. S. (2014). Qualitative research as living within/transforming complex power relations. *Qualitative Inquiry.*

Cannella, G. S., & Lincoln, Y. S. (2011). Ethics, research regulations, and critical social science. In N. K. Denzin & Y. S. Lincoln (Eds.), *The SAGE handbook of qualitative research* (4th ed. pp. 81–90). Thousand Oaks, CA: Sage.

Cannella, G. S., & Manuelito, K. (2008). Feminisms from unthought locations: Indigenous worldviews, marginalized feminisms, and revisioning an anticolonial social science. In N. K. Denzin, Y. S. Lincoln, & L. T. Smith (Eds), *Handbook of critical and indigenous methodologies* (pp. 45–59). Thousand Oaks, CA: Sage.

Cannella, G. S., & Miller, L. L. (2008). Constructing corporatist science: Reconstituting the soul of American higher education. *Cultural Studies ↔ Critical Methodologies, 8*(1), 24–38.

Cannella, G. S., Perez, M. S., & Pasque, P. (2015). (Eds.). *Critical qualitative research: Foundations and futures.* Walnut Creek, CA: Left Coast Press, Inc..

Collins, P. H. (2000). *Black feminist thought: Knowledge, consciousness, and the politics of* empowerment (2nd Ed.). New York: Routledge.

Deleuze, G. (1988). *Foucault.* Minneapolis: University of Minnesota Press.

Deleuze, G., & Guattari, F. (1977). *Anti-oedipus: Capitalism and schizophrenia.* Trans. R. Hurley, M. Seem, & H. R. Lane. New York: Penguin.

Deleuze, G., & Guattari, F. (1987). *A thousand plateaus: Capitalism and schizophrenia.* Trans. B. Massumi. Minneapolis: University of Minnesota Press.

Denzin, N. K., & Giardina, M. D. (2009). Qualitative inquiry and social justice: Toward a politics of hope. In N. K. Denzin & M. D. Giardina (Eds.), *Qualitative inquiry and social justice* (pp. 11–50). Walnut Creek, CA: Left Coast Press, Inc..

Dilts, A. (2010). *From 'entrepreneur of the self' to 'care of the self': Neoliberal governmentality and Foucault's ethics.* Chicago: Western Political Science Association 2010 Annual Meeting.

Eisenstein, Z. (1999). Constructing a theory of capitalist patriarchy and socialist feminism. *Critical Sociology, 25* (2/3), 196–217.

Felski, R. (1998). Images of the intellectual: From philosophy to cultural studies. *Continuum, 12* (2), 157–171.

Foucault, M. (1977). Preface. In G. Deleuze, & F. Guattari. (Eds.), *Anti-oedipus: Capitalism and schizophrenia* (pp. xi–xiv). Trans. R. Hurley, M. Seem, & H. R. Lane. New York: Penguin Group.

Foucault, M. (1982). The subject and power. In H. Dreyfus & P. Rabinow (Eds.), *Michel Foucault: Beyond structuralism and hermeneutics* (pp. 208–216). Chicago: University of Chicago Press.

Foucault, M. (1984). *The Foucault reader.* P. Rabinow (Ed.). New York: Pantheon.

Foucault, M. (1988). *Technologies of the self: A seminar with Michel Foucault.* L. H. Martin, H. Gutman, & P. H. Hutton (Eds.). Amherst: University of Massachusetts Press.

Foucault, M. (1997). *Michel Foucault: Ethics, subjectivity, and truth, 1954–1984, Vol. 1.* P. Rabinow (Ed.). New York: New York Press.

Foucault, M. (2003). *Society must be defended: Lectures at the College de France, 1975–76.* Trans. D. Macy. New York: Picador Palgrave Macmillan.

Foucault, M. (2008). *The birth of biopolitics: Lectures at the College de France, 1978–79.* Trans. G. Burchell. New York: Picador Palgrave Macmillan.

Goetsch, L. A. (2010). Open access starts with you. *Change Magazine, 42* (2), 50.

Kincheloe, J. L. (2008). Critical pedagogy and the knowledge wars of the twenty-first century. *International Journal of Critical Pedagogy, 1*(1), 1–22.

Klein, N. (2014). *This changes everything: Capitalism vs climate.* New York: Simon & Schuster.

Lemke, T. (2011). *Biopolitics: Medicine, technoscience, and health in the 21st century.* New York: New York University Press.

Lincoln, Y. S. (2010). Accountability, Texas-style. *21st Century Scholar.* Retrieved July 6, 2014, from 21centuryscholar.org/2010/09/09/accountability-texas-style-by-yvonna-lincoln/

Lincoln, Y. S. (2011). "A well-regulated faculty….": The coerciveness of accountability and other measures that abridge faculties' right to teach and research. *Cultural Studies ↔ Critical Methodologies, 11*(4), 369–372.

Lincoln, Y. S. (February, 2012a). Critical qualitative research and the corporatized university on a collision course: Reimagining faculty work and forms of resistance. Velma E. Schmidt Endowed Chair Lecture, College of Education, University of North Texas, Denton.

Lincoln, Y. S. (2012b). The political economy of publication: Marketing, commodification, and qualitative scholarly work. *Qualitative Health Research, 22*(11), 451–459.

Lincoln, Y. S., & Cannella, G. S. (2007). Ethics and the broader rethinking/reconceptualization of research as construct. In N. K. Denzin & M. D. Giardina (Eds.), *Ethical futures in qualitative research: Decolonizing the politics of knowledge* (pp. 67–84). Walnut Creek, CA: Left Coast Press, Inc.

Lincoln, Y. S., & Cannella, G. S. (2009). Ethics and the broader rethinking/reconceptualization of research as a construct. *Cultural Studies ↔ Critical Methodologies, 9* (2), 273–285.

Lorde, A. (1984). The master's tools will never dismantle the master's house. In *Sister outsider: Essays and speeches* (pp. 110–114). Berkeley, CA: Crossing Press.

McNay, L. (2009). Self as enterprise: Dilemmas of control and resistance in Foucault's *The Birth of Biopolitics. Theory, Culture & Society, 26*, 55–77.

Macey, D. (1993). *The lives of Michel Foucault.* New York: Vintage.

Marttila, T. (2013). *The culture of enterprise in neoliberalism: Specters of entrepreneurship.* New York: Routledge.

Oksala, J. (2005). *Foucault and freedom.* Cambridge, UK: Cambridge University Press.

Pinar, W. F. (2001). *The gender of racial politics and violence in America: Lynching, prison rape, & the crisis of masculinity.* New York: Peter Lang.

Rose, N. (1999). *Powers of freedom: Reframing political thought.* Cambridge, UK: Cambridge University Press.

Sawicki, J. (2013). Queer feminism: Cultivating ethical practices of freedom. *Foucault Studies, 16*, 74–87.

Sedgwick, E. (2003). *Touching feeling: Affect, pedagogy, performance.* Durham, NC: Duke University Press.

Slaughter, S., & Rhoades, G. (2004). *Academic capitalism and the new economy: Markets, state, and higher education.* Baltimore, MD: Johns Hopkins University Press.

Smith, L. T. (1999). *Decolonizing methodologies: Research and indigenous peoples.* London: Zed Books.

Thompson, K. (2003). Forms of resistance: Foucault on "tactical reversal and self-formation." *Continental Philosophy Review, 36*, 113–138.

Trujillo, C. (Ed.). (1998). *Living Chicana theory.* Berkeley, CA: Third Woman Press.

Von Werlhof, C. (2007). Capitalist patriarchy and the negation of matriarchy: The struggle for a 'deep' alternative. In S. Vaughan (Ed.), *Women and the gift economy: A radically different world view is possible* (pp. 139–153). Toronto: Inanna.

Winnubst, S. (2012). The queer thing about neoliberal pleasure: A Foucauldian warning. *Foucault Studies, 14*, 79–97.

Chapter 3

Practices for the "New" in the New Empiricisms, the New Materialisms, and Post Qualitative Inquiry

Elizabeth Adams St. Pierre

Several years ago I introduced the concept, *post qualitative inquiry* (St. Pierre, 2011a), to destabilize what I've called "conventional humanist qualitative inquiry," which I argue has become overdetermined by the publishing industry, university research courses, and journals and books that detail very carefully what it is and how to do it. As Law (2004) explained, "*particular* sets of rules and procedures may be questioned and debated, but the overall need for proper rules and procedures is not. It is taken for granted that these are necessary" (p. 5). To me, it is ironic that so much qualitative research has become formalized, precise, and methods-driven because it was invented in the 1980s (e.g., Denzin, 1989; Erickson, 1986; Lincoln & Guba, 1985) as an *interpretive* social science—drawing from the larger interpretive turn and, especially, from interpretive anthropology (e.g., Geertz, 1973)—to deliberately counter the methods-driven approach of positivist social science. Interpretive social science, unlike positivism, argues that method can't guarantee validity and that any "finding" is simply an interpretation which rests on other interpretations—"it's turtles all the way down" (Geertz, 1973, p. 29)—not on the Cartesian bedrock of uncontested truth.

Qualitative Inquiry and the Politics of Research edited by Norman K. Denzin and Michael D. Giardina, 75–95. © 2015 Left Coast Press, Inc. All rights reserved.

In education, in particular, the scientifically-based, evidence-based research movement initiated by the United States with the No Child Left Behind Act of 2001 (NCLB) contributed to the tightening up of the so-called emergent nature of qualitative methodology. In particular, NCLB created a new funding agency for educational research, the U.S. Institute of Education Sciences (note how easily education became a science), and its goal was to fund causal research using its gold standard, the randomized controlled trial, that supposedly proves beyond a doubt "what works" in schools, thereby shifting our focus—even in qualitative methodology—from interpretation and contingency to causation and final truth. As a result, we now have a great deal of positivist qualitative research, which is not surprising because, as Steinmetz (2005) noted, positivism is the "epistemological unconscious" of the social sciences, and 1980s qualitative methodology never did rid itself of positivist concepts like validity, bias, subjectivity (as in "subjectivity statements"), triangulation, coding data, audit trails, inter-rater reliability, and so on. The positivism always embedded in qualitative methodology now thrives. For example, I receive a steady flood of emails inviting me to learn how to code qualitative data using various software programs, a practice I argue is unthinkable in interpretive social science, much less "post" work. And I despair when doctoral students' response to questions about their dissertation research is something like, "I'm doing a case study" or "I'm doing an autoethnography" or "I'm doing an interview study." In other words, they respond with a "research design." When I ask them what theories they're thinking with in their studies, they seldom respond coherently. It appears they've studied some kind of stripped down methodology (or more accurately, they've learned some methods) but not epistemology or ontology. I believe this is a failure to teach, not necessarily a failure to learn.

Of course, the creeping control of Institutional Review Boards (IRB) that often don't understand qualitative methodology has contributed to its positivism by requiring researchers to follow bizarre practices such as signing your own consent form to do autoethnographic research.

But in 2014, the National Research Council (NRC) released a committee report (available free from the National Academy

Press website) that proposed revisions to the Common Rule. This report is sponsored not only by the National Research Council committee organized for the purpose but also by other prestigious national committees as well as the American Educational Research Association. In my reading of the report, it appears that much qualitative research will either be exempt from IRB review or expedited. This is certainly good news for qualitative researchers. Of course, we'll have to wait and see whether the proposed recommendations are included in the revision of the federal law, but if they are, they could eventually help loosen up the structure of qualitative research in the United States. Interestingly, I have already heard quite a bit of resistance to the proposed revisions from qualitative researchers, which is not surprising, given how quickly we accept current dominant, disciplinary structures as normal, necessary, and good.

But there is always resistance to the excess of power. Even as much educational research was taken over by the State Science Machine at the beginning of this century, thereby quantifying students and teachers as well as research methodology, others in the humanities and social sciences shifted from Enlightenment humanism's epistemological rage for knowledge that guides methods-driven qualitative methodology with all its "practices of formalization" (Pascale, 2011, p. 17) to the ontological—the nature of being—which I believe qualitative methodology mostly avoids. In conventional humanist qualitative methodology, to be is to know.

This new work has organized itself differently as affect theory (Gregg & Seigworth, 2010), thing theory (Brown, 2001), actor network theory (Latour, 2005), assemblage theory (De Landa, 2006), the new materialism (Coole & Frost, 2010), the new empiricism (Clough, 2009), and the posthuman (Braidotti, 2013). But I argue that poststructural theorists, including Derrida, Foucault, Lyotard, Baudrillard, and, especially, Deleuze and Guattari, very clearly addressed ontological issues and the material half a century ago. For example, last year I re-read with my doctoral students Foucault's *Archaeology of Knowledge* (1971/1972) and *The Order of Things* (1966/1970), and we found ontology and the material everywhere. And how could one say that Derrida, with his critique of *presence,* neglects the ontological, which explains why Kirby (2011) and Barad (2010) make good use of Derrida in their "new" work.

Much of the new empirical, new material, posthuman, post qualitative work uses the ontology of Deleuze and Guattari, who offer a constellation of imbricated concepts (e.g., *rhizome, assemblage, plane of consistency, refrain, diagram*) that enable a different ontology and their transcendental empiricism. Working with DeleuzoGuattarian concepts is not easy. For example, one can't understand a concept like *diagram* without understanding others it works with—*assemblage, abstract machine, plane of consistency, Body without Organs*—and they constantly introduce new concepts. In addition, a concept that is primary in one text, for example, *sense* in *Logic of Sense* (1969/1990), may not be used again.

We have been slow to take up Deleuze's and Deleuze and Guattari's ontology in the social sciences not only because, as Lyotard (1979/1984) noted, "we are stuck in the positivism of this or that discipline" (p. 41), but also because their work was translated into English later than other twentieth century French theorists'. Deleuze visited the United States only once, whereas Foucault and Derrida were frequent, popular lecturers, and translations of their work were quickly available. Most importantly, Deleuze and Guattari's work is deliberately ontological and difficult for those of us who've been so obsessed with knowledge projects that we've neglected to study ontology.

For those reasons, I believe this new empirical work that uses Deleuze and Guattari is difficult to think because we have to learn a new language that is incompatible with the ontological grids of intelligibility that structure humanist methodologies. And it's also difficult to do because there are no prescribed "methods" to follow or textbooks that offer, say, four handy research designs for new empirical research. If such a book were written, it would be contrary to the very image of thought Deleuze and Guattari created.

About method, Deleuze and Guattari (1980/1987) wrote that "a 'method' is the striated space of the *cogitatio universalis* and draws a path that must be followed from one point to another" (p. 377). In other words, the very idea of method forces one into a prescribed order of thought and practices that prohibits the experimental nature of transcendental empiricism. Method proscribes and prohibits. It controls and disciplines. Further, method always comes too late, is immediately out-of-date, and is therefore inadequate to the task at hand. But method not only can't keep up with events; more seriously, it prevents them from coming into existence. One might say that "method," as we think of it in the methodological individualism of conventional humanist qualitative methodology with its methods of data collection and methods of data analysis, *cannot be thought or done in new empirical inquiry.*

The most popular method of data collection in conventional humanist qualitative methodology is the face-to-face interview with its privileging of the authentic voice of the unique individual, the person, the human of humanism (for critiques, see St. Pierre, 2008, 2011b), but Deleuze and Guattari were not interested in the speaking subject; as Lecercle (2002) noted:

> The detailed study of an everyday discussion or telephone conversation yields trivial and uninteresting results, for such everyday exchanges are fully functional from the point of view of communication, and more often than not irenic [*sic*]. And they do have a point, to be reached and negotiated as swiftly as possible. . . . But there is hardly any novelty involved, even if (especially if?) the conversation becomes personal and garrulous. As a result, we have a series of utterances without interest . . . a static talking machine. (p. 199)

For Deleuze and Guattari, language used in conversation comes from the *order-words* of the *collective assemblage of enunciation*, the discursive relations of power that underlie the usage of a language and discipline thought and speech. What people say in ordinary conversation mostly echoes, repeats, dominant discourse.

Foucault, too, made it clear in his archaeological and genealogical analyses that he was not interested in the conscious, knowing, rational, intentional speaking subject with its confessional tendencies. Much like Deleuze and Guattari, he focused instead on what was "given to the speaking subject" (Foucault, 1971/1972, p. 46) in the anonymous murmur of the discursive formations from which speech emerges, from the order of things, the grid of intelligibility that pre-exists an "I" created by language, an "I" who, once created, falsely believes it exists ahead of language and can speak with individual intention. We social scientists who want to do this "new" work and also want to base our science on the voices of our research participants might remember Foucault's (1966/1970) project in *The Order of Things*:

> I tried to explore scientific discourse not from the point of view of the individuals who are speaking, nor from the point of view of the formal structures of what they are saying, but from the point of view of the rules that come into play in the very existence of such discourse: what conditions did Linnaeus (or Petty, or Arnauld) have to fulfill, not to make his discourse coherent and true in general, but to give it, at the time when it was written and accepted, value and practical application as scientific discourse. (p. xiv)

Those interested in the new empiricisms, especially in the post-human, must call into question the endless interviews that presume the humanist human, the *cogito*, who can know and speak the truth, who can *mean*. The onto-epistemological formation that celebrates the speech of the humanist human and assigns it pre-eminent value and practical application as scientific discourse is not the onto-epistemological formation of post-qualitative inquiry. For that reason, we should think, and should always have thought, twice before proposing research projects with, for example, an awkward combination of an interview study and a Foucaultian genealogy or a rhizo-analysis of interview data, projects that indicate ontological confusion.

What this comes down to, I believe, is that if one wants to move toward this new empirical, new material, posthuman, post qualitative inquiry, one must begin anew with little "methodological" help—with no new empirical methods textbooks that describe research designs (recipes) and structuring practices that explain where to begin and what to do next and then next. In other words, to do this work, one must give up that sacred validating concept *systematicity* which is supposed to guarantee that qualitative methodology is rigorous science and not, say, journalism. To me, systematicity smacks of scientism. But Lyotard (1979/1984) explained the work of the postmodern artist or writer decades ago, and his description suits the work of new empirical inquiry:

> The text he writes, the work he produces [is] not in principle governed by preestablished rules, and [it] cannot be judged according to a determining judgment, by applying familiar categories to the text or to the work. Those rules and categories are what the work of art itself is looking for. The artist and the writer, then, are working without rules in order to formulate the rules of what *will have been done*. Hence the fact that work and text have the character of an *event*; hence also, they always come too late for their author, or, what amounts to the same thing, their being put into work, their realization (*mise en oeuvre*) always begins too soon. (p. 81)

Interestingly, we seemed not to have understood Lyotard's (and other poststructuralists') comments about the postmodern as we diligently tried, for too long, to mix postmodern scholarship and methods-driven research. But the new empirical work rings alarms that method can only be described after the fact; it can neither guide a research project nor guarantee its validity. In fact, the new empiricist might well argue that attempting to follow a given research method will likely foreclose possibilities for the "new." The new empiricist researcher, then, is on her own, inventing inquiry in the doing.

But who wants to work so hard? Who wants to have to invent new empiricist inquiry and invent it anew for every study? A counter-question might be how we came to think we didn't have to? Eisner (quoted in Saks, 1996) helped us think about difficult work and taking risks when he wrote that we should "work at the edge of incompetence" (p. 412), and Foucault (1984/1985) offered the following encouragement:

> As to those for whom to work hard, to begin and begin again, to attempt and be mistaken, to go back and rework everything from top to bottom, and still find reason to hesitate from one step to the next—as to those, in short, for whom to work in the midst of uncertainty and apprehension is tantamount to failure, all I can say is that clearly we are not from the same planet. (p. 7)

Surely, this is the pleasure of scholarship, this not-knowing and, as Derrida (1980/1987) wrote, "knowing how not to be there and how to be strong for not being there right away. Knowing how not to deliver on command, how to wait and make wait" (p. 191). Perhaps not knowing and waiting describe the *style* of the new empirical researcher.

To sum up before moving on, I argue that much conventional humanist qualitative methodology, invented in the 1980s, was never able to make the interpretive turn and shed its positivist heritage. Further, the demands of scientifically-based and evidence-based research at the beginning of the twenty-first century restored and reinstalled positivism throughout the social sciences, especially in education. But qualitative research has always been another Enlightenment knowledge project focused on methodology and the production of knowledge. Typically, its structure and formalized practices have not only been weak epistemologically— e.g., when researchers avoid theorizing and only "find themes in the data"—but also ontologically. What this means is that qualitative methodology seems to stand outside epistemology and ontology. We all know this work. Given that, it is very difficult for one well-trained in this kind of qualitative methodology to make this ontological turn toward new empirical, new material, posthuman, post qualitative inquiry.

What Is *New* in New Empirical Inquiry?

As I wrote earlier, I introduced the concept *post qualitative inquiry* in 2011 to encourage researchers to move past 1980s qualitative methodology, much of which I believe has been overtaken by positivism. In 2013, Patti Lather and I edited a special issue of the *International Journal of Qualitative Studies in Education* on post qualitative inquiry. In 2014, Alecia Jackson and I edited a special issue of *Qualitative Inquiry* on qualitative data analysis after coding. Alecia Jackson, Lisa Mazzei, and I are currently editing a special issue of *Cultural Studies ↔ Critical Methodologies* on the new empiricisms/new materialisms. Other special issues of journals as well as recent edited and authored books announce that scholars are taking up the challenges of new inquiry.

But in reviewing manuscripts submitted to journals in which authors claim to be doing new empirical, new material, posthuman, and post qualitative work, I find myself hard-pressed to see what's "new" about much of it. It's as if people try but can't quite make the ontological turn, and I surely understand that. I'm not sure I can either. Like MacLure (2013), I believe the "shock" of working "within a materialist ontology has not yet been fully felt" (p. 663).

But whenever I'm interested in something new—to me, at least—I teach a course about it so my smart students can help me think. Two years ago I taught a new doctoral seminar, the "New Empiricisms and the New Materialisms," and last year I taught a doctoral seminar I developed in 2003 called "Post Qualitative Research," the content of which has changed significantly over the years. In both courses, my students and I struggled to think about how to "do" social science inquiry differently if one thinks with those scholars we call poststructuralists as well as those writing more recently about the ontological turn. What would be new and different about that work? And where would one *begin* to do this "new" kind of inquiry? It's all well and good to follow Deleuze and Guattari and say "begin in the middle"—even if that's probably the best advice—but what does that look like? And how does a *new* researcher even *know* whether something is "new" and "different"? And how different do you have to be to be "new"? Do you have to invent an entire methodology or can you just struggle with what's pressing in your own project? More practically, how can you increase your odds of doing something "new"?

With those questions in mind, I first review how two theorists who critiqued humanist ontology, Foucault and Deleuze, described the "new." Then, given their descriptions, I offer in the next section a few practices I think might be useful in getting us unstuck from conventional humanist qualitative methodology whose structure traps us and prevents us from making that ontological turn and moving toward the "new."

I begin with Foucault (1971/1972), who wrote early in his career in the *Archaeology of Knowledge* that "it is not easy to say something new." Nonetheless, we know Foucault did say quite a few new things. He also said in an interview two years before he died at 54, "I worked like a dog all my life" (Foucault, 1982, p. 131) because his project was *his own transformation*. He said, "Do you think I have worked like that all those years to say the same thing and not to be changed"? This is interesting, isn't it?

Foucault's warning us not only that doing something new is very hard work but that scholarly work is personal and not just academic. I agree and tell my students that if they're working hard to read Foucault and Deleuze and Guattari and Derrida and Barad and Baudrillard and Bennett and Bergson and Spinoza, they *will be changed,* and they can't go back. Thus, my advice to them is that if they're especially fond of themselves as they are, they'd best avoid reading this literature on the "posts" and on ontology and go to the movies or mow their yards instead.

Rajchman (2008), discussing Deleuze's (1986/1988) book on Foucault, explained that, for Foucault, the new is "not at all what is in fashion, but rather what we cannot yet see or say in what is happening in us just because it is not already contained in the ... given [structures] that govern what we can think" (p. 89). We can't see the new because of the structures of the present, and we have no language yet to say it. Almost a hundred years ago, Whitehead (1925) wrote that pre-existing structures normalize our thinking and produce "minds in a groove" (p. 197), but experimentation can help us move out of the grooves of the normal and self-evident. For Foucault, Rajchman (2008) explained, the new is "a pragmatic experimental matter, something we must actually do for which there precedes no determination, no model, no 'we,' not even an 'I'" (p. 89). Again, there is no model (no method, no research design, nor an "I") that exists ahead of experimental work that pushes toward the new and different.

Deleuze also believed that it is only in a practical and experimental engagement with the world that we can create something new, because "the new is an outside that exists within this world, and as such it must be constructed" (O'Sullivan & Zepke, 2008, p. 2). For Deleuze (1968/1994), "the new, with its power of beginning and beginning again, remains forever new, just as the established was always established from the outset, even if a certain amount of empirical time was necessary for this to be recognized" (p. 136). So it may take some time to distinguish the new that is always becoming from the established that is. For this reason, the new can't easily be *recognized* because it is outside our grids of intelligibility.

Most importantly, using language from major, structuring discourses (e.g., systematic science, methodological positivism, the solipsism of the Cartesian knower) is dangerous because the language of those discourses does not work after the ontological turn (e.g., see MacLure, 2013; St. Pierre, in press). Major, dominant language describes what is recognizable, already captured, disciplined, and normalized—what *is*—not what is immanent but not yet, what could be becoming if we were able to resist the present and think/do it. That is Deleuze and Guattari's (1991/1994) famous challenge: "We lack creation. *We lack resistance to the present*" (p. 108). Foucault's (1982) challenge in regard to the present and, especially, to subjectivity is similar—"to refuse what we are" (p. 216). In both cases, we must refuse *order-words* that enforce the present and, in this case, methodological order-words like method, systematicity, transparency, representation, validity, objectivity, and so on. These words force us into *is*.

Practices for the "New"

Why is it so difficult to take up the new empirical inquiry? As I've studied the manuscripts I review in which authors claim to be doing post qualitative work but aren't and as I work with students who struggle to do something different, I've realized they often make the mistake of beginning with conventional humanist qualitative methodology. That is, they begin in a humanist instead of a posthumanist ontology. For example, they might include in the theoretical sections of their papers a smart discussion of DeleuzoGuattarian concepts they say informed their research, but then they proceed to describe their projects as conventional humanist qualitative studies using the ontological assumptions, language, and practices of that methodology. In effect, they simply drop one or two Deleuzian concepts into a qualitative study and, of course, the ontologies are incommensurable. I don't see how these confused projects can produce anything "new."

Why does this happen? I believe that in too much social science research we chiefly teach methodology, having separated it from epistemology and ontology, thereby reducing inquiry to method and research design. Hence, we have methods-driven research that mostly repeats what is recognizable, what is already known.

What we fail to teach is epistemology and ontology. We fail to teach theory. Why? I believe it's easier to teach methods than theory. It's easier to teach, say, five research designs than DeleuzoGuattarian ontology, which is very difficult to understand. Lecercle (2002) wrote that it took him thirty years to begin to understand Deleuze's (1969/1990) book, *The Logic of Sense.* And you have to read Deleuze and Guattari's (1980/1987) long book, *A Thousand Plateaus: Capitalism and Schizophrenia*, which is not logically sequential, before you're ready to read it. Again, who wants to work so hard?

Out of this, I have begun to recommend some specific practices that might increase our odds of accomplishing something "new" in new empirical, new material, posthuman, post qualitative inquiry: refusing qualitative methodology, reading, beginning with theory/concepts instead of methodology, and trusting ourselves in not knowing. Of course, these practices are not radical but are, I would argue, age-old practices of solid scholarship.

First practice: Refuse qualitative methodology.

My key recommendation for those who want to attempt new empirical inquiry is to forego methods-driven research of any kind and instead read theory. Thus, my first "practice for the new" in new empirical inquiry is to leave conventional humanist qualitative methodology behind, to refuse it. Those of us who've learned it too well will just have to try to forget it. We should remember that we invented this methodology in the 1980s—we made it up—and it's not sacred. It's simply one approach among others, and we can't take it too seriously. The ontology of this methodology retains the human/nonhuman, word/thing, representation/the real distinctions, which are unintelligible in new empirical inquiry in which "the separation between subject and object, thought and matter, words and things, is an illusion of language" (Lecercle, 2002, p. 27).

I believe qualitative methodology is a trap for those who want to do new empirical inquiry. It traps us when we drop a concept like the rhizome or assemblage from Deleuze and Guattari's experimental ontology into the structure of a humanist interview study that privileges the ontology of the "speaking subject." It traps us when we retain concepts like *data* and *subjectivity* that are not thinkable in the same way, if at all, in an experimental ontology. In other words, using a concept from one ontology in another just doesn't work. Those of us interested in the "post" theories spent many years deconstructing the concepts of conventional humanist qualitative inquiry (e.g., interview, data, voice, validity, reflexivity) and working its ruins (St. Pierre & Pillow, 2000), but we remained trapped in those ruins, I believe, by not attending to ontological issues. I suggest we do something different from the beginning.

Second practice: Read, read, read.

I advise my students who want to do new empirical, new material, posthuman, post qualitative work to shift their focus from methodology to onto-epistemology. Reading a few of the many texts that introduce qualitative, quantitative, and mixed methods research is sufficient. I encourage them to spend their time reading and re-reading scholars who have written about onto-epistemology for centuries. This reading is the true pleasure of our lives as academics, and I believe inquiry begins by reading what Foucault (1971/1972) called the "already said" (p. 25) that may well be "new" for us and give us language and strategies to think and do our own "new."

I tell my doctoral students, "No one can read for you. You have to do it yourself. And those who read a lot can always tell when others don't." I tell them that the most voracious readers know that the image of thought within which we comfortably think and live may well be demolished by reading the next book or journal article and that, at some point, "shock to thought" (Massumi, 2002) is our desire. I caution them about reading too many books they understand. I encourage them to organize reading groups to read books that are too hard to read and to set up what I call "reading management strategies" (see St. Pierre, 2014) to keep track of their reading so they can use it later for writing.

I tell them that if they keep reading, if they *read and read and read*, if they let the words and concepts wash over them, they will, indeed, begin to put them to work in their everyday lives. They will understand what Foucault meant when he said we have to give up the "we" and the "I." They'll understand why Deleuze refused the personal pronouns. They will no longer believe or live the human/nonhuman binary.

At some point, they begin to understand the impossibility of "human subjects research" as conceived by conventional humanist qualitative methodology and Institutional Review Boards. Instead, they grapple with theory—for example, with Deleuze and Guattari's (1980/1987) shocking ontological statement, "There is no longer a tripartite division between a field of reality (the world) and a field of representation (the book) and a field of subjectivity (the author). Rather, an assemblage established connections between certain multiplicities drawn from each of these orders" (p. 23). In this flattened ontology, human bodies, other living bodies, objects, language, representations, concepts like revenge, values like goodness, dreams, green, a memory, the weather, five-o'clock in the afternoon, and the not-yet are mixed, entangled on the surface. There is no depth in this ontology as there is in structuralism and phenomenology. The human is no longer prior to language, method, and the world; in fact, the human being of humanism is no longer intelligible.

It is impossible to think humanist "human subjects research" when, to simplify Deleuze and Guattari, we are always *assemblages* that are not stable entities that can be broken down into distinct component parts and made to mean, but rather that are, something like machines, constantly territorializing and deterritorializing—becoming. Importantly, assemblages do not imply interiority but exteriority, so we would not ask what an assemblage *is* or what parts it contains but rather with what it connects, what it plugs into. Again, human being is not independent and self-contained but mixed with everything else on the surface. We cannot separate out the human subject in posthuman, new empirical, new material, post qualitative inquiry. Our responsibility is no longer to the privileged human but to the assemblage, which is always more-than-human and always becoming. In this age of the anthropocene, responsibility assumes its full meaning.

This brief description gestures toward the ontological image of thought that guides the new empiricisms and displaces humanist qualitative inquiry. At the heart of this ontology are very different understandings of *language* and *human being* that we must account for. Once those two concepts in humanist ontology are shattered, we no doubt flounder; but it is from that not knowing that the "new" might emerge. Of course, the poststructuralists told us this decades ago, but, stuck in the groove of humanist qualitative methodology, we somehow mostly ignored that profound rupture.

I surely did not understand Deleuze's and Deleuze and Guattari's work together when I first read it early in my doctoral studies—not in a university course but on my own—nor do I "understand" it now. Nonetheless, the image of thought enabled by their concepts like haecceity, assemblage, and Bodies without Organs stuck with me, ruining conventional humanist qualitative methodology from the start. I am grateful I read Deleuze and Guattari, Butler, Spivak, Foucault, Baudrillard, Lyotard, Derrida, and others we call "post" before I was over-trained in humanist qualitative methodology, before its methods-driven structure took over my thought and practices.

Third practice: Begin with theory/concepts.

So if, for example, a doctoral student has avoided learning too much conventional humanist qualitative methodology and has, instead, studied onto-epistemology, what might she do next for her dissertation research? She may well panic because her classmates may have begun their studies by following the clear instructions of the plethora of books and journal articles that describe the "research process" in quantitative, qualitative, or mixed methods studies. They have a well-trod path to follow.

To repeat, I advise students not to begin with methodology but with theory(ies) or a concept or several related concepts they've identified in their reading that helps them think about whatever they're interested in thinking about (e.g., reluctant readers, the quantified student, marriage, happiness) (see, e.g., Jackson & Mazzei, 2012). If a student is interested in Foucault's theory of *power*, she should read everything he wrote about power as well as secondary sources and critiques. If she's interested in Derrida's *deconstruction*, she should read (almost) everything he wrote about deconstruction as well as secondary sources and critique. The same would hold for Lyotard's *paralogy*, and Butler's *gender*, Barad's *entanglement*, Bennett's *vital matter*, Deleuze and Guattari's *assemblage*, and so on. In Deleuze and Guattari's work, one concept is seldom enough because their concepts are entangled, just like their ontology. The point here is that sustained and "careful reading" (Butler, 1995) is required and brings some measure of confidence and expertise so that students understand why they cannot carelessly mix ontologies.

To repeat, the theory(ies) and/or the concept(s), then, instead of a pre-determined research method, guides the study. From among many concepts, the researcher chooses those that help her think about whatever she wants to think about. She plugs concepts into the world to see how they work. If she's studied the theory in depth, good questions to ask when confused might be "What would Foucault do?" "Would Derrida code data?" "Would Lyotard use the concept triangulation?" And the best thing to do when confused is to go back to the texts and re-read the theory, to plunge into the words of scholars who inspire.

I am not especially concerned with classifying or labeling this kind of inquiry, because post-method, "after method" (Law, 2004), every study will be different and unclassifiable, which will no doubt make some uneasy: "What *is* this study?" We will have to train ourselves not to look for prescribed method, familiar practices of formalization, and tortured systematicity in this work.

Of practical concern, of course, is how scholars doing this post-qualitative, new empirical, new material, posthuman work think about Institutional Review Boards and "human subjects." I expect, however, that the recommendations of the National Research Council committee, mentioned earlier, will be used to revise the Common Rule and may well obviate the need for human subjects review for most conventional humanist qualitative methodology and especially for posthuman studies. Appendix B of the NRC report (2014) described the types of studies it recommends be exempt from review:

> Benign interactions or interventions that involve methodologies that are very familiar to people in everyday life and in which verbal, behavioral, or physiological responses would be the research data being collected (e.g., educational tests, surveys, focus groups, interviews, fieldwork or "participant observation," and

similar procedures; and sociolinguistic studies, simulation studies; games, markets, negotiations, voting; individual or group decision making; studies of educational processes, teaching, and learning; studies of social perception and judgment; personal, achievement, and ability tests, and role playing involving routine activities or tasks under different scenarios and that do not in and of themselves introduce or heighten physical pain or psychological discomfort). (p. 156)

Further, these exemptions "would not be limited to adults" (p. 156). These recommendations will produce a sea change in social science research and remove us from the thrall of Institutional Review Boards. The rest is up to us.

Fourth practice: Trust yourself and get to work.

The fourth practice I recommend to students, after they've given up qualitative methodology, have read and read and read, and have found theory(ies) and/or concept(s) to guide their inquiry, is to trust themselves. I encourage them to just put to work the practices the theory/concept enables—we might call these *conceptual practices* (Harding, 2007; Smith, 1990)—to do the next thing experimental ontology enables them to think and do. These practices may be quite familiar, what we do when we want to explore anything. For example, we read, we write, we talk with other people, we observe what's going on around us. We may make a movie, paint a picture, run a marathon—who knows? In the name of positivist social science, which permeates conventional humanist qualitative methodology, we have, as the recommendations for revisions to the Common Rule acknowledge, overdetermined, over-formalized, systematized, and scientized some everyday practices out of all proportion to legitimate them as "scientific," but we have completely ignored others. In conventional humanist qualitative methodology, we've mostly reduced research practices to two "methods of data collection," interviews and observations, though I doubt the concepts "data" or "methods of data collection" are thinkable in new empirical inquiry in which the human has never been separate from "data," outside it, so she could "collect" it. The language of qualitative methodology surely traps us.

The point here is that ordinary practices like talking with and observing people don't have to be scientized and elevated to the status of "the interview" and "the observation." I'm interested in all the other practices we neglect to disclose. For example, when I'm deep into a project and stuck, I go for a walk or weed my garden and inevitably get unstuck. I have called this the "physicality of theorizing" (St. Pierre, 1997, p. 184), so I suppose I could call *walking* and *weeding* research practices—but why would I? And, surely, we could name *reading* a research practice, but we don't—we call it the "literature review." I'm very interested in conceptual practices concepts like diagram, Bodies without Organs, entanglement, vital matter enable. What would one *do* if one were thinking and living with those concepts? I've noticed that some of my students are particularly drawn to music in their new empirical work.

My strongest recommendation is that we not try to force our new empirical, new material, posthuman, post qualitative studies into the structure of conventional humanist qualitative methodology. I can't imagine how it could fit. Instead of beginning with methodology, I recommend putting the concepts and theories of experimental ontology to work using the conceptual practices that are appropriate for a particular study. If we've done our reading, I wager we cannot *not* put it to work. It will have transformed us—we cannot think and live without it. *We will be living it.*

As Foucault and Deleuze explained, the "new" is already in our lives, but repetition of the same cannot create it. We have to make it. It is in the experimental moment of *not* knowing what to do next because we are *not* driven by method and methodology that we might push through the grooves of the given and the self-evident toward the new and different in our work and lives. Method, then, will always come at the end, too late, when we think back about what we did and why and what we might have done instead and will try next time.

References

Barad, K. (2010). Quantum entanglements and hauntological relations of inheritance: Dis/continuities, spacetime infoldings, and justice-to-come. *Derrida Today, 3(2)*, 240–268.

Braidotti, R. (2013). *The posthuman.* Cambridge, UK: Polity Press.

Brown, B. (2001). Thing theory. *Critical Inquiry, 28*(1), 1–22.

Butler, J. (1995). For a careful reading. In S. Benhabib, J. Butler, D. Cornell & N. Fraser (Eds.), *Feminist contentions: A philosophical exchange* (pp. 127–143). New York: Routledge.

Clough, P. T. (2009). The new empiricism: Affect and sociological method. *European Journal of Social Theory, 12*(1), 43–61.

Coole, D., & Frost, S. (Eds.). (2010). *New materialisms: Ontology, agency, and politics.* Durham, NC: Duke University Press.

De Landa, M. (2006). *A new philosophy of society: Assemblage theory and social complexity.* New York: Continuum.

Deleuze, G. (1988). *Foucault.* S. Hand, Trans. Minneapolis: University of Minnesota Press. (Original work published 1986.)

Deleuze, G. (1990). *The logic of sense.* C. V. Boundas (Ed.); M. Lester (Trans.). New York: Columbia University Press. (Original work published 1969.)

Deleuze, G. (1994). Difference and repetition. P. Patton (Trans.). New York: Columbia University Press. (Original work published 1968.)

Deleuze, G., & Guattari, F. (1987). *A thousand plateaus: Capitalism and schizophrenia.* B. Massumi (Trans.). Minneapolis: University of Minnesota Press. (Original work published 1980.)

Deleuze, G., & Guattari, F. (1994). *What is philosophy?* H. Tomlinson & G. Burchell (Trans.). New York: Columbia University Press. (Original work published 1991.)

Denzin, N. K. (1989). *Interpretive interactionism.* Newbury Park, CA: Sage.

Derrida, J. (1987). *The post card: From Socrates to Freud and beyond.* A. Bass (Trans.). Chicago: University of Chicago Press. (Original work published 1980.)

Elliot E., in Saks, A. L. (1996). *Viewpoints*: Should novels count as dissertations in education? *Research in the Teaching of English, 30* (4), 403–427.

Erickson, F. (1986). Qualitative methods in research on teaching. In M. C. Wittrock (Ed.), *Handbook of research on teaching* (3rd ed., pp. 119–161). New York: Macmillan.

Foucault, M. (1970). *The order of things: An archaeology of the human sciences.* A. M. S. Smith (Trans). New York: Vintage Books. (Original work published 1966.)

Foucault, M. (1972). *The archaeology of knowledge and the discourse on language.* A. M. S. Smith (Trans.). New York: Pantheon Books. (Original work published 1971.)

Foucault, M. (1982). The subject and power. In H. L. Dreyfus & P. Rabinow, *Michel Foucault: Beyond structuralism and hermeneutics* (2nd ed., pp. 208–226). Chicago: University of Chicago Press.

Foucault, M. (1985). *The history of sexuality. Volume 2. The use of pleasure.* R. Hurley (Trans.). New York: Vintage Books. (Original work published 1984.)

Geertz, C. (1973). *The interpretation of cultures: Selected essays.* New York: Basic Books.

Gregg, M., & Seigworth, G. J. (Eds.). (2010). *The affect theory reader.* Durham, NC: Duke University Press.

Harding, S. (2007). Feminist standpoints. In S. N. Hesse-Biber (Ed.), *Handbook of feminist research: Theory and praxis* (pp. 45–69). Thousand Oaks, CA: Sage.

Jackson, A. Y., & Mazzei L. A. (2012). *Thinking with theory in qualitative research: Viewing data across multiple perspectives.* London: Routledge.

Kirby, V. (2011). *Quantum anthropologies: Life at large.* Durham, NC: Duke University Press.

Latour, B. (2005). *Reassembling the social: An introduction to actor-network-theory.* Oxford, UK: Oxford University Press.

Law, J. (2004). *After method: Mess in social science research.* London: Routledge.

Lecercle, J-J. (2002). *Deleuze and language.* New York: Palgrave Macmillan.

Lincoln, Y. S., & Guba, E. G. (1985). *Naturalistic inquiry.* Newbury Park, CA: Sage.

Lyotard, J-F. (1984). *The postmodern condition: A report on knowledge.* G. Bennington & B. Massumi (Trans.). Minneapolis: University of Minnesota Press. (Original work published 1979.)

MacLure, M. (2013). Researching without representation? Language and materiality in post-qualitative methodology. *International Journal of Qualitative Studies in Education, 26*(6), 658–667.

Massumi, B. (Ed.). (2002). *A shock to thought: Expression after Deleuze and Guattari.* London: Routledge.

National Research Council. (2014). *Proposed Revisions to the Common Rule for the Protection of Human Subjects in the Behavioral and Social Sciences.* Committee on Revisions to the Common Rule for the Protection of Human Subjects in Research in the Behavioral and Social Sciences. Board on Behavioral, Cognitive, and Sensory Sciences, Committee on National Statistics, Division of Behavioral and Social Sciences and Education. Washington, DC: The National Academies Press.

O'Sullivan, S., & Zepke, S. (2008). Introduction: The problem of the new. In S. O'Sullivan & S. Zepke (Eds.), *Deleuze, Guattari and the production of the new* (pp. 1–10). New York: Continuum.

Pascale, C-M. (2011). *Cartographies of knowledge: Exploring qualitative epistemologies.* Los Angeles: Sage.

Rajchman, J. (1985). *Michel Foucault: The freedom of philosophy.* New York: Columbia University Press.

Rajchman, J. (2008). A portrait of Deleuze-Foucault. In S. O'Sullivan & S. Zepke (Eds.), *Deleuze, Guattari and the production of the new* (pp. 80–90). New York: Continuum.

Saks, A. L. (1996). Viewpoints: Should novels count as dissertations in education. *Research in the Teaching of English, 30,* 403–427.

Smith, D. (1990). *The conceptual practices of power: A feminist sociology of knowledge.* Toronto: University of Toronto Press.

Steinmetz, G. (2005). The epistemological unconscious of U.S. sociology and the transition to post-Fordism: The case of historical sociology. In J. Adams, E.S. Clemens & A.S. Orloff (Eds.), *Remaking modernity: Politics, history, sociology* (pp. 109–157). Durham, NC: Duke University Press.

St. Pierre, E. A. (1997). Methodology in the fold and the irruption of transgressive data. *International Journal of Qualitative Studies in Education, 10*(2), 175–189.

St. Pierre, E. A. (2008). Decentering voice in qualitative inquiry. In A.Y. Jackson & L. Mazzei (Eds.), *Voice in qualitative inquiry: Challenging conventional, interpretive, and critical conceptions* (pp. 221–236). New York: Routledge.

St. Pierre, E. A. (2011a). Post qualitative research: The critique and the coming after. In N. K. Denzin & Y. S. Lincoln (Eds.), *Sage handbook of qualitative inquiry* (4th ed., pp. 611–635). Los Angeles: Sage.

St. Pierre, E. A. (2011b). Refusing human being in humanist qualitative inquiry. In N. K. Denzin & M. D. Giardina (Eds.), *Qualitative inquiry and the global crisis* (pp. 40–55). Walnut Creek, CA: Left Coast Press, Inc.

St. Pierre, E. A. (2014). An always already absent collaboration. *Cultural Studies ↔ Critical Methodologies, 14*(4), 374–379.

St. Pierre, E. A. (in press). Deleuze and Guattari's language for new empirical inquiry. *Educational Philosophy and Theory.*

St. Pierre, E. A., & Pillow, W. S. (Eds.). (2000). Working the ruins: Feminist poststructural theory and methods in education. New York: Routledge.

Whitehead, A. N. (1925). *Science and the modern world* [Lowell Lectures, 1925]. New York: The Free Press.

Chapter 4

The Work of Thought and the Politics of Research

(Post)qualitative Research

Patti Lather

My father retired from 36 years of school teaching around the same time as Johnny Carson was stepping down from late night television, and now I find myself retiring from 36 years of teaching as David Letterman announces he will step aside. The generational sweep in late night television says something about "time to go" and whatever meaning might be made of this time, this place in the realm of qualitative research.

While my title indicates some sweeping programmatic vision for the field, I will use the occasion of this talk to first go small in terms of my own retirement project on sports and schooling modeled after Walter Benjamin's *Arcades Project* (1999). I will conclude by abstracting out from that project whatever grand programmatic pronouncements I cannot help myself from making.

I begin by framing the work of thought and the politics of research with my own story of generational shifts in feminist theory. My journey moves across the ideology critique in which I was trained as a doctoral student through the deconstruction that stopped me in my tracks for a few years in the mid-80s to, quite recently, the post-post or ontological turn with which I am

Qualitative Inquiry and the Politics of Research edited by Norman K. Denzin and Michael D. Giardina, 97–117. © 2015 Left Coast Press, Inc. All rights reserved.

presently wrestling. In this, I use Gayatri Spivak's (2012) cautionary definition of theory as what we call philosophy today; something we can hide behind; something to help us read the world; something to help us change the world; something we use in bullying.

Generational Thinking: The Ontological Turn

Deborah Britzman (1999) has written of what she calls "thoughts awaiting thinkers," and that has been my experience of, again, trying to take yet one more turn, of once more scouring bibliographies to keep moving into the becoming of feminist theory and methodology, of once more undoing what I thought I could not think without, to draw on Spivak's insight into the difficulties of such movement.

There have been continuities of concern across my work: thinking within and beyond various interdisciplines into narrations of methodology, epistemologically travelling from getting smart to getting lost, politically attuned to feminism across its shifts and turns and multiplicities. Quite some time ago, I broke with an intellectual landscape of philosophical Masters and Mistresses who focused on dialectics with its oppositions, sequential negations, progress narratives, and varied idealisms, including the heroic researcher. At the beginning of my scholarly life in the late 1970s, we called it "socialist feminism," which in the late-1980s segued into "poststructural feminism," bookended by my initial confusion with Donna Haraway's "I'd rather be a cyborg than a goddess" (I was a goddess girl myself at that time) and by my much more immediate and even relieved grasp of Judith Butler's early 90s troubling of gender. Of late, I have begun dating a different set of theorists. Here, for want, perhaps, of better terms, my interest is the non-foundational materialist approaches that Rosi Braidotti (2005) has appropriated from Deleuze and Guattari and termed "feminist post-postmodernism." Such "becomings" of feminist theory and methodology are embodied and embedded breakings of canonized processes. My interest is in the implications of these dynamics for the "passing on" of the moments and movements of feminist thought and practice from one generation to the next.

One way to frame all of this is in the possible displacement of Judith Butler by Karen Barad in feminist theory where the fifteen-year span from Judith Butler's 1993 *Bodies That Matter* to Karen Barad's 2007 *Meeting the Universe Half-Way* has opened up much talk about posthuman theory and methodology. While Butler's conceptual grammar provided performativity in identity/self formation as a kind of corporeal matter, the matter of matter has exploded well beyond the body and the subject, well beyond even human life, well beyond even the posthuman (Bogost, 2012). "Do rocks have consciousness?" asks Australian anthropologist Elizabeth Povenelli (2011) in some neo-materialist way that is not about pre-critical animism but rather intra-relational co-constitutive two way traffic between things and language and interpretation. This could be compressed into tracing the move from "radical constructivism" to "posthuman intra-relationality" where ontology and epistemology collapse into one another. Shifting from objects to assemblages and from proliferating and competing paradigms to meta-method across disciplines,[1] Barad (2007), drawing from feminist science studies, queer theory and Niels Bohr's "philosophy-physics" (2012a, p. 11), puts forward the concept of agential realism out of her strong critique of social constructivism. The hoped for result is to materialize methodologies that cross the humanities and the sciences toward more intra-active, webbed, and networked understandings of the messy and fluid objects of the world.

Given the "high interdisciplinarity" (Braidotti, 2013, p. 58) at work, these methodological perspectives range across what Braidotti lists as deconstructive, post-anthropocentric, post-constructionist, the new empiricism, critical posthumanism, new feminist materialism, "after" actor-network theory (Fenwick & Edwards, 2010), new science studies, neo-Foucauldian bio-politics, and the neo-humanism of global post-colonialism. Regardless of disciplinary terminology, these moves encompass both scientific and technological complexity with implications for theories of the subject,[2] political economy, and governmentalities. They, as well, call for research practices that are situated and accountable, "views from somewhere" as Donna Haraway (1988) said almost thirty years ago in her call for situated knowledges.

What is new here is the ontological insistence on the weight of the material and a relational ontology that transverses binaries. Particularly important is the immanence of agency, a key rethinking of this question of agency that has haunted all of deconstruction (Hey, 2006) and where the gravitational pull of humanism is especially strong (Barad, 2012b, p. 54). "Natureculture" (Haraway's term) becomes one word; matter becomes generative; intra-action becomes the motor of a distributed agency where Barad's (2007) "agential realism" breaks with Butler's more subject-centered identity and social/psychic entanglements. What Barad (2007) terms the "agential qualities of matter" rise to the fore in a move that portends a more productive engagement across the human and natural sciences where "an objectivity of actualization and realization" becomes a perpetual flow and "matter matters" (van der Tuin & Dolphijn, 2010, p. 169).

All about networks and "assemblages," Barad is the Queen of this space.[3] Her project of rethinking the humanist subject maps onto Deleuze[4] and the networked virtualities of becoming. Her work helps us see how liberal humanism, always the temptation, gets reinscribed as reflexivity materializes "the authentic and really real" via an "intentional and conscious" researcher (Mazzei, 2013, p. 778). Lisa Mazzei terms this the way the "knowing humanist subject… lingers in some post-structuralist analysis" (p. 778). Barad 's ontological focus interrupts this temptation more than Butler's tendency to re-center the humanist subject given her epistemological focus and the constitutive force she gives to language and culture (Kirby, 2002), what some have called a "failed materialism" that re-inscribes the cultural and linguistic turns (Dolphijn & van der Tuin, 2012).[5]

In learning to better understand how we get "pulled back into the same old humanist orbits" (Barad, 2012b, p. 54), the key is our entanglement in a time when the epistemological tide has ebbed and object oriented philosophies are in ascendance. A sort of post-posthumanism brackets human actors in a neo-decentering of the subject. This produces a "flattened relationship" (Bogost, 2012, p. 5; Mazzei, 2013, p. 778) rather than a hierarchy, an entangled becoming out of intra-action and diffraction that works as a difference driven analytic. This is where I want to install myself via a self-narrative of memory that is "not already coded" in reflexive or autoethnographic ways, but, rather, a "thinking through the body" (p. 782) of the experience of feminist research in post-post times.

One of Walter Benjamin's favorite sayings during long slow walks was "tiens tiens!" by which he meant, "Stop so we can think!" (Eiland & Jennings, 2014, p. 373). I want now to take a slow walk so that I can think my way into an empirical project toward which I have been moving perhaps all my life.

Sports and Schooling Project

> *I'm not actually bothered about my chances of being fulfilled in real terms... It's just the will to fulfillment that blazes, that's indestructible.*
>
> (Roland Barthes, *A Lover's Discourse*, emphasis in the original)

This section will provide an "expose" or current state of a so far virtual project that might remain that way. Using Walter Benjamin's *Arcades Project* as a model toward a book about sports and U.S. secondary schooling, I unpack the aggregate of materials collected as well as the "theoretical armature" (Eiland & Jennings, 2014, p. 483) and methodological principles involved. The goal is to proceed configuratively, like an archaeological dig, into a montage book that functions as a social memory and historical index of an under-appreciated aspect of the shaping of teacher hiring practices in American schooling, what I call the 6,000 pound question of whether we hire teachers or coaches.

The pile of my collected materials includes a recent *NY Times* article (April 25) on the Andy Warhol show at the Queens Museum that writes of how "the wealth of supporting material" provides a "deep context" through "miracles of archive diving" on the part of the curators through "ephemera" that evoke what it meant for Warhol to be caught "when two damaged decades were slamming together" (p. C25).

This evokes my sense of Walter Benjamin in the Bibliotheque Nationale de Paris the last ten years of his life as he assembled his "convolutes" or files. Spreading it out on my living room floor, I organized the archive I have been assembling for almost ten years now. Files range across news reports on the historical configuration around football in the United States, including, importantly, concussion fears.[6] The "situational mapping" (Clarke, 2005) of my files includes the Penn State sex abuse scandal and the window it provides into big time college sports; models of international schooling that deal quite differently with the question of sports; charter schools, school reform, and the scandals and critiques thereof; the quest for teaching excellence and the big money and bad science involved; cheerleading; stories of high school coaching, including those of my father and brothers; and media and pop culture sports stories that have opened up a world of which I would not otherwise have made much note. This includes my deep addiction to the television show, *Friday Night Lights*, as a historical index into the small town Americana out of whence I came, and most recently the documentary film, *We Could Be King*, about the merging due to budget cuts of two bitter rival Philadelphia school football teams. This latter maps onto oral history research on the race dynamics involved in football at desegregated schools in Mississippi that troubles "the myth of sports as the great racial unifier in the South" (Adams & Adams, 2014; Lee Bell, *Now Can We Talk?* 2013).

An annual ranking of U.S. high schools (Mathews, 2014) argues "a shift in high school culture" where "something significant is happening... for many of our highest performing high schools, football is no longer part of the culture."[7] Although both sports and solid academics are present in some few places, "the national trend" is that "more schools [are] adopting the European and Asian models of few sports but lots of serious studying." Most visible on this front is the recent work of Amanda Ripley. Her book, *The Smartest Kids in the World and How They Got that Way* (2013), compares "no sports curriculums" as the norm in Finland, Germany, South Korea, and Poland with American norms. Ripley intersects an ingenious sample of exchange students and Programme for International Student Assessment (PISA) test results to address how sports are embedded in an "unholy alliance" (p. 119) in U.S. high school culture compared to other "superpower" countries.[8] Her work was a cover story for the October 2013 issue of *The Atlantic*, entitled "How Sports Are Ruining High School: The Real Reason U.S. Students are Falling

Behind." In an unexpected way, the upshot of all of this appears to be an underscoring of a recent focus on the costs of economic inequality.[9]

Rather than feeling like I am too late to the ball, this is the "perfect storm" that impels me forward in studying the weight of sports on U.S. secondary schooling. Not to make too much of it, post-angel as I am, it does evoke Benjamin's Angel of History with eyes wide open, blown backwards by history into a future where what was once impossible to think, the end of school-sponsored football, is newly thinkable.

In terms of the theory I draw on, more than a reading history, such an archival listing explores an ideascape as part of a wider geography of knowledge that shapes a field and my work. One can map this generative influence via the new conceptual grammar provided by Karen Barad and the spread of her ideas. Elizabeth de Freitas (2014), a math educator, is but one example. Rethinking the relationship between the quantitative and the qualitative out of the new materialism, her focus is what she terms "an objective unruliness" (p. 5). Unpacking how "a new kind of empiricism may be at our doorstep," de Freitas looks at quantity and chance in exploring "a new burgeoning relationship" between the quantitative and the qualitative (p. 12). She moves beyond mechanistic and determinist theories of matter toward a re-inscription of quantification, calculation, and measurement built on an understanding of indeterminacy and chance as ontological. Privileging difference and multiplicity, she "centres affect and aesthetics as engines of activity" (p. 2). Her bibliography leans heavily on Barad, Latour, and Deleuze, with smatterings of feminist, queer, and science studies and a sort of Foucauldian attention to obscure thinkers of "ancient little book[s]" that foreshadow the quantitative aspects of our (post)modernity.[10] "The social life of quantitative methods" (p. 6) and a "re-animated" take on the quantitative start looking like generative tools in the question of method in digital times. Here "following the objects" leads the analysis toward an appreciation of "quantitative multiplicity—the intrinsic difference at the heart of all processes of becoming" (p. 11). Digital navigation, large data mining methods, and new visualization software provide us access to networks of associations that are based, not on structure, but on particulars as traces that allow us to "follow the dynamic aggregate as it grows… [where] interaction [is] an undulating generative network" (p. 12). Drawing heavily from Latour, de Freitas argues that the quantitative, too, has "an unscripted future."

Well, I think you can appreciate that I have surely ventured into unknown territory here. To draw on the Deleuzean language of Brian Massumi (2002), perhaps this space is a "pure virtuality, barely thinkable" where the present practice of qualitative research carries the seeds of its own collapse and where a virtual metalogic is called for in thinking within and beyond it.[11] What this means theory-wise in my own project includes what it means for a project to be "a work projected out ahead," as Barthes says in *The Preparation of the Novel* (2011, p. 165), a project "of throwing something out ahead of you, from springboard to springboard" (p. 149) where young scholars like de Freitas can spring me way beyond my comfort zone.

Finally, in terms of methodological principles to guide me in this project, I have found Hillevi Lenz-Taguchi's 2012 essay on diffractive analysis particularly useful for its critique of reflexivity as caught up in discursivity at the expense of materiality. The former reflects the same, the latter differentiates. Using both Butler and Barad to make her argument (p. 270), interfering with the data, she elaborates on the intra-relation and co-constitutiveness of data and analysis. What one sees is how the "bodymind" of the researcher becomes "a space of transit" (p. 272), a reading "with" the data that is an embodied engagement toward a thinking otherwise that enacts "*intervention* and *invention*; *responsibility* and *ethics*" (p. 278, emphasis in the original). Here a new kind of object comes to attention, an object "pulled out of shape by its framings" and, equally importantly, "framings pulled out of shape by the object" (Rifkin, 2003). This challenges who you think you are as a researcher in a way that holds promise for advancing the critical edge of practice.

I tried this in my very short essay on the Penn State sex abuse scandal where I did, in fact, feel my way into a different analytic space that was not particularly comfortable (Lather, 2012). To enact what unexpected angle a "becoming feminist" diffractive analysis might provide, I found myself "*intra-acting* from within" in a way immanent to a particular event where we interrupt our usual "*perceptual style* and *habits of seeing*" (Jackson & Mazzei, 2012, p. 134, emphasis in the original). My move was toward a "becoming with" in ways not already coded, where a researcher actively resists his or her own interpretation toward a "different subjectivity… a subject position not previously experienced" (p. 133). What was materialized in this "intra-relational" method was a fraught space where I became a fragile thinker as this nexus of issues pushed me places I was not sure I wanted to go in exploding the container into which sports and sexual abuse have been bottled up. All of this harbors caution for my inquiry into sports and schools. Poised on retirement's edge, hoping to produce something that will make use of all my skills and interests and contribute to how we might think in different ways about schools, sports, and what feminist analysis is and might become in such a space, this may be a stretch that takes me to the beyond of myself in thinking my way into the (post)qualitative.[12]

Comingling old and new practices in complex ways, such work materializes vibrant and robust dynamic interplays, intermixings, distributed contingencies, and productive tensions. Here, in Hillevi's words again, "new events of thinking get materialized…, [d]ata get lived in new ways," and researchers undo themselves into creative thinkers in assemblage with one another. Exploring the production of new terms of "being-acting-feeling together" that are community based, community sustaining, and community serving (MacLellan & Talpalaru, 2012), a new culture of method is materialized out of breaking methodological routine by "taking the risk of a new relationality" (Berlant, in Davis & Sarlin, 2008).

I'm not sure what this new relationality means. For me, who has almost always worked alone, with the notable exception of Chris Smithies in the study of women and HIV/AIDS (Lather & Smithies, 1997), I am especially struck with the teamwork model of this recent work. While I always felt I materialized a textual network via relational practices of, perhaps, over-quoting, this generation models, in Hillevi's words, needing "others in order to displace and unhinge" their own understandings (2013, p. 639). While I have been part of many a reading group, this is a "companionship" in scholarly production that results in a collective process as a very social enterprise that breaks with the privatizing and individualizing model in which I grew up. My new project provides an opportunity to break this aloneness in interviewing my brothers and other family members, transcribing my father, and perhaps following up with the sort of folks who have volunteered to work with me, including the many school teachers I have had in my classes who say "study my school" if I want to see these dynamics in action. This would surely break my usual lone ranger working habits and materialize a more collaborative assemblage of thinkers thinking our way into the (post)qualitative.[13]

Cloud Gate: Becoming (Post)qualitative

New work always involves objections to the old, but these objections are really relevant only to the new.

(Donald Judd, 1965)

My title is taken from the Cloud Gate sculpture in Chicago that inspires a kind of thinking about what is becoming in spaces of inbetweenness. In a not unusual move for me, turning to art practices to address whatever the post-qualitative might mean, the artist Donald Judd's thoughts on sculpture gesture toward how to think the new. Judd says of new work that "there hasn't been enough time and work to see limits," but it is "a space to move into" where its "characteristics are bound to develop" and where it can "be only what it is now which means that if it changes a great deal, it will be something else." Like Judd's new forms of art, it will have preliminaries and beginnings and "as if" moments of coming into being rather than the "set forms" of conventional qualitative research. It will be "as powerful as it can be thought to be," hopefully interesting, "intense, clear and powerful," producing "strange objects," perhaps, in being "not diluted by an inherited format."[14]

An additional art model, the Cloud Gate sculpture by Indian-born British artist Anish Kapoor in Chicago, as well spurs a kind of thinking about what is becoming. A "feasible method" had to be sought out for its stainless steel surface inspired by liquid mercury that distorts and twists what it reflects. The Cloud Gate sculpture blurs "the boundary between the limit and the limitless… evokes immateriality and the spiritual... occupies an illusory space... [and] explores the theme of ambiguity and 'inbetweenness.'" It is designed to demand interaction and limit viewers to a partial view, challenging perception "in a disorienting multiplicative manner that intensifies the experience" (Wikipedia).

These thoughts on sculpture suggest that a blueprint for post-qualitative might be materialized out of mutated dominant practices, through a convergence of intensity and emergence. Here practice and objects of a field are redefined and reconfigured. In excess of intersectionality in attending to multi-directionalities, posthuman bodies, intra-actional networks, contingency, non-mastery and incalculables, issues are taken on of messy conceptual labor, difference, otherness, and disparity. The move is towards glimmers of alternative understandings and practices that give coherence and imaginary to what is possible after the methodological positivism that has taken up too much of our time and attention since governmental incursion into scientific method.[15] The "positivist qualitative" dominant unleashed by "best practices" and "scaling up" with calls for procedural transparency, handmaiden to the state sorts of policy usefulness and consequent fundabilities, evidence-based this and that, and systematicities that reduce the wild profusion to the too rational-technical: all of this positivist qualitative work subsumes the "infinite" variety of interpretive research approaches. This surely includes the "mixed signals" (Yanow & Schwartz-Shea, 2014, p. 433) across three NSF funded workshops from 2003 to 2009 and mixed methods discussions that are, more than not, covers for positivist qualitative work.[16]

In contrast, the post-qualitative has to do with undoing. The passage of qualitative research beyond itself moves it deeper into complication and accountability to complexity and the political value of not being so sure (Lather, 2007). No more a progressive development, a replacing of one thing by another, any more than cubism replaced impressionism (Iversen & Melville, 2010, p. 192), the move is toward a research imaginary that finds shape and standards in what we are making in its name. This includes practices that no longer have such a hold on us that we struggle with ghosts as terms collapse.

The models that make the change begin to take shape in the exemplars I have probed over the last few years as well as in the sketch of my own work that I have offered here today as an interesting case to think with. I would also include the efforts I have been reviewing across a variety of qualitative journals and conferences as necessary fits and starts or hybrids of the old and the new, not unlike my 1991 *Getting Smart* that was a transitional hybrid of post-marxism and post-structuralism. In our contemporary post-post moment, "the post-qualitative" often takes the form of what used to be called "experimental" writing, sometimes along auto-ethnographic lines that re-inscribe the humanist subject. While representing what we are trying to get over, these are practices we don't know how to do without, mixed message texts not unlike *Getting Smart* that had me doing and undoing myself from one page to the next, riddled with contradictions in moving toward the new. But one example is my insistent hanging on to praxis without rethinking agency and the subject.

Other efforts I see that reinscribe what we are trying to get over include refusing fieldwork in a turn to the text, but this is hardly new. Neither is angst in fieldwork new, either epistemologically in terms of how we know or ontologically in terms of what we try to know. Refusing to put "the other" under our gaze is not new. Laurel Richardson turned some time ago from looking at the other to looking at herself as part of the auto-ethnographic turn in the name of ethics. A keen sense of the limits of our knowing, usually rendered as the confessional tale (van Maanen, 1988) is not new. Experimental writing in the social sciences is not new. There is even a book by that title from anthropology angst in its mid-1980s post-colonial moment (Marcus & Fischer, 1986). Too often in such efforts, into the vacuum of "the other under the microscope" comes the self, and while this self is in process and becoming and performing, it too often looks little different from the individual self of phenomenology.

Here affect theory might provide some direction as it troubles "the liberal culture of true feeling" (Berlant, 2011, p. 65) that is so sentimentally present in much of the qualitative research about the "vulnerable ethnographer" (Behar, 1996) and autoethnography. To interrupt the drama of the self, Berlant articulates a Raymond Williams "structure of feeling" that is refracted in shared historical time. Bespeaking a shared nervous system in this time of surviving neo-liberalism, Berlant terms this "a desubjective queerness" (p. 18) that is not so much internal self-involvement mired in narcissism as a sort of counter-affect that works against the "inflated poetic interiority" (p. 157) of a liberal investment in emotional authenticity, what Berlant terms "the demand for a feeling fix" (p. 176) that is a kind of "noisy affectivity."

Berlant's interest, as is mine, is in a postspectacular dedramatized story, a deflationary aesthetic that works at an ontological level to point to the insecurity of knowing. Calling on Agamben's "inoperative community," this is a non-relation that performs the impasse and the limitation of what feelings can do. Working out of a fatigue with affective inflation and resulting intensities, Berlant's counter affect positions feeling as just one nodal point among many and not the most important. The rescuing researcher is displaced in the transition from less heroic practices (Britzman, 2009) to a place where "a brush with solidarity" might be the best we can hope for in the present "bruising" affectsphere of "what is already not working" (Berlant, 2011, p. 263). Instead of a voice of masterful, individual authority, it does what Ronell (2010) calls "partnering up with the questioning other" in order to disrupt any settled places in our work.

Writing the post-qualitative and materializing practices that do not yet exist might be inspired by cultural events such as the documentary, "The Act of Killing." Recently nominated for an Academy Award, this film interviews the leaders of Indonesian death squads active in the mid-60s. Having them re-enact their now too-long-in-the-past-to-be-prosecuted killings, a multilayered participatory design unfolds as a member check unlike any I have ever seen. Allowing the killers to see themselves on their own terms, through a sort of "drama therapy" (LaSalle, 2013) of repeated viewings and enactments, the filmmaker plays with fire in exposing a regime of impunity out of the actors' own vanities, love of gangster movies, and everyone's necessary complicities. The film was shown in Indonesia and, by some reports, has transformed its sense of history in a truth and reconciliation sort of format. Delivering hard truths, the filmmaker has produced something devastating that you don't get to not see.

In sum, there is much to be said about the work of thought and the politics of research, including how the crisis of neoliberalism requires an ontological insurrection of a praxis from below, what Antonio Negri calls the "centrality of common praxis," a practical response within networked culture (2007, p. 64). This calls for a kind of participatory research on steroids, "doing research according to a logic of immersion, of situating ourselves inside the present, always starting from below where there is no outside" (pp. 63–64). Negri calls this "*joint-research*" (italics in the original) that "creates outlooks of struggle" by focusing on the commonalities of bodies and the desire for a future democracy, where networks of constitutive learners "no longer speak of taking power, but rather of *making power*" (p. 71, emphasis in the original).[17] Perhaps this instantiates Barad's call for an "iteratively reconfigured and enfolded" past and future "through the world's ongoing intra-activity" (Barad, 2012b).

Conclusion: Ontologizing the Remains

Diffraction… does not traffic in a temporality of the new…. [It is] a matter of inheritance and indebtedness to the past as well as the future.

(Barad, 2012a)

My interest in this chapter has been the development of a post-qualitative imaginary and its implications for empirical work. In addressing the thought to which all of this tends, I think what I am asking for is some framing along the lines of—hey, we are all in this together of figuring out what "post-qualitative " space looks like and here is my effort as it relates to other such efforts. We are not out here by ourselves. What can be abstracted from such efforts by way of a methodology that can move us away from the theories and practices whose grip on us we are trying to break?

It feels to me like the moment of attachment and detachment when those of us trained in ideology critique moved into deconstruction.[18] What had to be let go of? Of what could we/would we not let go? What continues to haunt the (be)coming methodology, a methodology defined as "applied ontology and epistemology" (Yanow & Schwedke Shea, 2014, p. xvi)?

In *Getting Lost* (Lather, 2007, pp. 104–105), in a chapter entitled "Applied Derrida," I delineated the shift from ideology critique to deconstruction as a movement away from the Enlightenment project that offers a knowable empirical and historical presence in contrast to the ontological uncertainty of deconstruction, from known unknowns to unknown knowns, to quote from Donald Rumsfeld (whom I never expected to quote).[19] "If such a thing exists," Derrida writes, over and over again, marking the indeterminacy that is the "originary complication" of a deconstruction that is not an unmasking but a keeping open, alive, loose, on guard against itself. Here troubling language as a transparent medium undercuts universal categories and a romanticized individual subject. Other necessary losses include the innocence and righteousness of the knower with his or her self-nominated "educative" role, intentional agencies of reason and will, fixities of identity, margins and centers, and, perhaps hardest to give up, the authority of what we know and how we know it. Thrust out of innocent knowingness by the post, we have been destabilized in paradoxes of necessarily complicit practices and proliferating differences where ways of knowing became an "archive of windows," a study of the histories of enframing with a focus on the staging of truthfulness. Perplexed by design, we moved from getting smart to getting lost as a matter of ethics and politics.

Now, in the post-post in what Barad terms the "ethico-onto-epistemological" (2012b), we can hardly recognize ourselves. Located as we are in neither "conventional humanistic qualitative research" (St. Pierre, 2011) nor the deconstructive variant that, perhaps, was a transition into this differently ontological space, we are still struggling with deconstructive troublings of a certain praxis of salvation narratives, consciousness raising, and a romance of the humanist subject and agency. And so we arrive at this point in the "becoming" of the (post)qualitative, at the question of how we ontologize what remains in the next generation of qualitative inquiry as we collectively imagine sustainable possible futures via new thought and present-based practices of everyday life.

Notes

1 George Marcus (2009) defines "meta-method" as that which rethinks and experiments with standard practices, moving beyond current scripts and their conventional situating of inquiry.

2 Post-post theories of the subject are called, variously, the Deleuzean subject (van der Tuin & Dolphijn, 2010, p. 164), the post-humanist subject (Braidotti, 2013), and the larval subject caught between the virtual and the actual (Bryant, 2006).

3 As Bruno Latour is "Prince of Networks," according to Graham Harman's 2009 book.

4 Barad talks much of the "dynamic and reiterative re-workings of Butler and Foucault" in her work (2012a, p. 12), but, without being exhaustive, I could find only one citation of Deleuze (his book on Foucault, 1988). See her 2003 *Signs* essay where she critiques Foucault for his passive theory of matter and puts a posthuman twist on Butler's theory of performativity.

5 Butler is referred to as "the epitome of linguisticism" who continues to "feed the dualism" in her new work (Dolphijn & van der Tuin, 2012, p. 114). An effort to "rescue" Butler for the new materialism is Kirby, 2006. An early critique is Fraser, 2002.

6 NBC Nightly News, January 31, 2014: regarding "organized football," 40% of parents will discourage their kids from playing. "I would not let my son play football" (Obama). Youth enrollment down 10%. NFL is being compared to having the blinders of Big Tobacco in 1960's. School districts are afraid of law suits.

7 In Mathews's list of top ten schools, one was without a football team in 1998, seven in 2014. This is linked to the lack of significant gains in average math and reading achievement among seventeen-year-olds in the past three decades. Although the top 10% lists 2,000 schools, with 82% "still" having football teams, non-football schools are at the top of the list.

8 PISA has its critics. See Meyer and Benavot, 2013.

9 *Capitalism in the Twenty-First Century* by the French "soft Marxist" economist, Thomas Piketty (2014), is an unexpected best-seller with its argument that inequality is structural and best thwarted by progressives taxation to limit the concentration of wealth that is destroying democracy.

10 What I particularly appreciate about de Freitas's 2014 AERA conference paper is how it exceeds its form in a kind of spill-over of vitality. She has "sections to be included in longer paper" at the end; she concludes with provocations about her own efforts "to tap into speculative arts-based forays into big data" that she does not have time to go into, while announcing how she finds these forays "disturbing" and "I'm not quite sure how to make sense of them." This announces work to come for which I can hardly wait.

11 This is a gloss on Kaufman (1998) who draws on Brian Massumi who draws on Gilles Deleuze regarding the collapse of capitalism in the face of the blurring between peace and war in current interventional efforts around the globe (p. 9).

12 Childers, Rhee, and Daza (2013) have theorized "promiscuous feminism" as a space for such work that, on the surface, has little to do with feminism. Barad says she frequently is asked, "'Since your work is not about women or gender, what does it have to do with feminism?' My answer, of course, was: 'Everything'" (2012b).

13 Additionally, Sara Childers has dissertation research that includes data on a school with a "no sports curriculum," and I have names jotted down of people I met on airplanes and conferences who have volunteered their schools for a study of "do we hire teachers or coaches?"

14 This phrasing has been adapted from Donald Judd's 1965 essay, "Specific Objects," on how to get clear of old forms in new work in painting and sculpture.

15 That such governmental incursion has by no means ended is evidenced by recent efforts (FIRST Act, H.R. 4186) to use NSF reauthorization to cut social, behavioral, and economic funding unless the NSF can justify how its funding serves "the national interest" (AERA, March 2014).

16 For a report on the 2003 workshop, see Ragin, Nagel, and White, 2004. For a report on the 2005 workshop, see Lamont and White, 2009, or www.nsf.gov/sbe/ses/soc/ISSQR_workshop_rpt.pdf. For the 2009 workshop, see www.ipia.utah.edu/imps/

17 An example of this is *On the Run: Fugitive Life in an American City*, by Alice Goffman (2014, University of Chicago Press), an intense, immersive, participatory ethnography of life in a low-income neighborhood of Philadelphia and the systems of surveillance and control that permeate lives and destroy relationships, families, and neighborhoods.

18 I remember Jane Kenway, for example, remarking at some conference that she had expected she would always do ideology critique. While I was glad enough to leave the strictures of Marxism, I think I thought I would be a social constructionist forever.

19 This is from the recent Errol Morris documentary, "The Unknown Known," about truth, power, and the Iraq War. A. O. Scott reviewed the film for the *New York Times*, characterizing it as "a probing and unsettling inquiry into the recent political and military history of the United States, but it is also a bracing and invigorating philosophical skirmish."

References

Adams, N., & Adams J. (2014). 'We all came together on the football field': Unpacking the blissful clarity of a popular Southern sports story. In W. Reynolds (Ed.), *Critical studies of Southern place: A reader* (pp. 337–347). New York: Peter Lang.

AERA speaks out against unprecedented cuts to NSF social science funding. (March 2014).

American Educational Research Association. Retrieved April 28, 2014, from www.aera.net/Newsroom/AERAHighlightsE-newsletter/AERAHighlightsMarch2014/peaksOutAgainstUnprecedentedCutstoNSFSocialScienceFunding/tabid/15416/Default.aspx

Barad, K. (2003). Posthumanist performativity: Toward an understanding of how matter comes to matter. *Signs, 28*(3), 801–831.

Barad, K. (2007) *Meeting the universe half-way*. Durham, NC: Duke University Press.

Barad, K. (2012a) Intra-active entanglements: An interview with Karen Barad. *Kvinder, Kon and Forskning NR, 1–2*, 10–23.

Barad, K. (2012b) Matter feels, converses, suffers, desires, yearns, and remembers: Interview with Karen Barad. In R. Dolphijn & I. van der Tuin (Eds.), *New materialism: Interviews and cartographies* (pp. 48–70). Ann Arbor, MI: New Humanities Press.

Barthes, R. (1978). *Lover's discourse: Fragments* (Trans. R. Howard). New York: Hill and Wang.

Barthes, R. (2011). *The preparation of the novel* (Trans. K. Briggs). New York: Columbia University Press.

Behar, R. (1996). *The vulnerable observer: Ethnography that breaks your heart*. Boston, MA: Beacon Press.

Bell, L. (2013). *Now can we talk?* Video. New York: Teachers College Press.

Benjamin, W. (1968/1940). Theses on the philosophy of history. In H. Arendt (Ed.), *Illuminations* (pp. 253–264). New York: Schocken Books.

Benjamin, W. (1999). *The arcades project* (Trans. H. Eiland and K. McLaughlin on the Basis of the German Volume, R. Tiedemann (Ed.). Cambridge, MA: Harvard University Press.

Berlant, L. (2011). *Cruel optimism*. Durham, NC: Duke University Press.

Bogost, I. (2012). *Alien phenomenology, or, What it's like to be a thing*. Minneapolis: University of Minnesota Press.

Braidotti, R. (2005) A critical genealogy of feminist post-postmodernism. *Australian Feminist Studies, 29*(47), 169–180.

Braidotti, R. (2009). Introduction: Learning from the future. *Australian Feminist Studies, 24*(59), 3–9.

Braidotta, R. (2013) *The posthuman*. Cambridge, UK: Polity Press.

Britzman, D. (1999). Thoughts awaiting thinkers: Group psychology and educational life. *International Journal of Leadership in Education, 2*(4), 313–335.

Britzman, D. (2009). *The very thought of education*. Albany, NY: SUNY Press.

Bryant, L. (2006). Larval subjects [blog]. www.larvalsubjects.wordpress.com

Butler, J. (1993). *Bodies that matter*. New York: Routledge.

Childers, S., Rhee, J. E., & Daza, S. (2013). Promiscuous (use of) feminist methdologies: The dirty theory and messy practice of educational research beyond gender. *Qualitative Studies in Education, 26*(5), 507–523.

Clarke, A. (2005). *Situational analysis: Grounding theorizing after the postmodern turn*. Thousand Oaks, CA: Sage.

Davis, H., & Sarlin, P. (2008). "On the risk of a new relationality": An interview with Lauren Berlant and Michael Hardt. *Reviews in Cultural Theory*. Retrieved August 23, 2012, from reviewsinculture.com/special-issue/review1.html

Deleuze, G. (1988). *Foucault*. Minneapolis: University of Minnesota Press.

De Freitas, E. (2014). New materialist ontologies of chance: Quantitative methods and qualitative becoming. Paper presented at the annual convention of the American Educational Research Association, Philadelphia, April 3–7.

Dolphijn, R., & van der Tuin, I. (2012). *New materialism: Interviews and cartographies*. Ann Arbor, MI: New Humanities Press.

Eiland, H., & Jennings, M. W. (2014). *Walter Benjamin: A critical life*. Cambridge, MA: Harvard University Press.

Fenwick, T., & Edwards, R. (2010). *Actor-Network Theory and education*. London: Routledge.

Fraser, M. (2002). What is the matter of feminist criticism? *Economy and Society, 31*(4), 606–625.

Haraway, D. (1988). Situated knowledges. *Feminist Studies, 14*(3), 575–599.

Harman, G. (2009). *Prince of networks: Bruno Latour and metaphysics*. Melbourne: re:press.

Hey, V. (2006). The politics of performative resignification: Translating Judith Butler's theoretical discourse and its potential for a sociology of education. *British Journal of Sociology of Education, 27*(4), 439–457.

Iversen, M., & Melville, S. (2010). *Writing art history: Disciplinary departures*. Chicago: University of Chicago Press.

Jackson, A., & Mazzei, L. (2012) *Thinking with theory in qualitative research*. London: Routledge.

Judd, D. (1965). Specific objects, *Arts Yearbook 8.*

Kaufman, E. (1998). Introduction. In E. Kaufman & K. Heller (Eds.), *Deleuze and Guattari: New mappings in politics, philosophy and culture* (pp. 3–13). Minneapolis: University of Minnesota Press.

Kirby, V. (2002). When all that is solid melts into language: Judith Butler and the question of matter. *International Journal of Sexuality and Gender Studies, 7*(4), 265–280.

Kirby, V. (2006). *Judith Butler: Live theory.* London: Continuum.

Lamont, M., & White, P. (2009). *Workshop on interdisciplinary standards for systematic qualitative research.* Washington DC: National Science Foundation.

Lasalle, M. (2013, Aug. 8). 'The act of killing' review: Amazing documentary. *San Francisco Chronicle.* Retrieved February 10, 2015, from www.sfchronicle.com/entertainment/article/The-Act-of-Killing-review-Amazing-documentary-4717557.php?t=f8c50aaf2547b02379

Lather, P. (1991). *Getting smart: Feminist research and pedagogy with/in the postmodern.* New York: Routledge.

Lather, P. (2007). *Getting lost: Feminist efforts toward a double(d) science.* Albany, New York: SUNY Press.

Lather, P. (2012). Becoming feminist: An untimely meditation on football. *Cultural Studies ↔ Critical Methodology, 12*(4), 357–360.

Lather, P. (2013). An intellectual autobiography: The return of the (feminist) subject? In M. B. Weaver-Hightower & C. Skelton (Eds.), *Leaders in gender and education* (pp. 117–128). Rotterdam: Sense.

Lather, P., & Smithies, C. (1997). *Troubling the angels: Women living with HIV/AIDS.* Boulder CO: Westview Press.

Lenz-Taguchi, J. (2012). A diffractive and Deleuzean approach to analyzing interview data. *Journal of Feminist Theory, 13*(3), 265–281.

MacLellan, M., & Talpalaru, M. (2012). Remaking the commons. *Reviews in Cultural Theory.* Retrieved on August 22, 2012, from reviewsinculture.com/special-issue/

Marcus, G. (2009). Introduction. In J. Faubion & G. Marcus (Eds.), *Fieldwork is not what it used to be* (pp. 1–31). Ithaca, NY: Cornell University Press.

Marcus, G., & Fisher, R. (1986). *Anthropology as cultural critique: An experimental moment in the human sciences.* Chicago: University of Chicago Press.

Massumi, B. (2002). *Parables for the virtual: Movement, affect, sensation.* Durham, NC: Duke University Press.

Mathews, J. (April 7, 2014). At many leading schools, football fails to make the cut. *Washington Post.*

Mazzei, L. (2013). Materialist mappings of knowing in being: Researchers constituted in the production of knowledge. *Gender and Education*, *25*(6), 776–785.

Meyer, H., & Benavot, A. (Eds.) (2013). *PISA, power, and policy: The emergence of global educational governance*. New York: Oxford University Press.

Negri, A. (2007). Logic and theory of inquiry: Militant praxis as subject and as episteme. In S. Shukaitis & D. Graeber, with E. Biddle (Eds.), *Constituent imagination: Militant investigations/ collective theorization* (pp. 62–72). Oakland, CA: AK Press.

Piketty, T. (2014). *Capital in the twenty-first century* (Trans. A. Goldhammer). Cambridge, MA: Harvard University Press.

Povenilli, E. (2011). *Economies of abandonment: Social belonging and endurance in late liberalism*. Durham, NC: Duke University Press.

Ragin, C., Nagel, J., & White, P. (2004). *Report of the workshop on scientific foundations of qualitative research*. Arlington, VA: National Science Foundation.

Rifkin, A. (2003). Inventing recollection. In P. Bowman (Ed.), *Interrogating cultural studies* (pp. 101–124) London: Pluto Press.

Ripley, A. (2013). *The smartest kids in the world and how they got that way*. New York: Simon and Schuster.

Ripley, A. (2013, October). The case against high school sports. *The Atlantic*. Retrieved February 10, 2015, from www.theatlantic.com/magazine/archive/2013/10/the-case-against-high-school-sports/309447/

Ronel, A. (2010). *Fighting theory*. Urbana: University of Illinois Press.

Spivak, G. (2012). *An aesthetic education in the era of globalization*. Cambridge, MA: Harvard University Press.

St. Pierre, E. (2011). Post-qualitative research: The critique and the coming after. In N. Denzin & Y. Lincoln (Eds.), *The SAGE handbook of qualitative research, 4/e* (pp. 611–635). Thousand Oaks, CA: Sage.

Van der Tuin, R., &, Dolphijn, R. (2010). The transversality of new materialism. *Women: A Cultural Review*, *21*(2), 153–171.

Van Maanen, J. (1988). *Tales of the field*. Chicago: University of Chicago Press.

Yanow, D., & Schwartz-Shea, P. (Eds.) (2014). *Interpretation and method: Empirical research methods and the interpretive turn*, 2/e. Armonk, NY: M. E. Sharpe.

Chapter 5

Qualitative Data Analysis 2.0

Developments, Trends, Challenges

Uwe Flick

Introduction

At the celebrations for the 50th anniversary of the Institute for Advanced Studies in Vienna, Austria, the science researcher Helga Novotny (2014) mentioned that it is dangerous for an academic institution to become fifty. According to Novotny, the first crisis starts when an institution becomes twenty, because then the memories of the founding fathers and mothers start to fade. First adaptations to changing circumstances become necessary after the period of expansion is finished (p. 16). In 2014, the institution of the International Congress of Qualitative Inquiry celebrated its tenth anniversary. This means it is currently in full swing of growing up rather than of growing old. Founding fathers and mothers are still fully involved in this development. Expansions on the levels of participation (growing numbers of participants and more and more countries being involved) and of issues to be dealt with are still a leading momentum.

A look on the history of these congresses as reflecting the history of qualitative inquiry reveals a development along a number of themes (see Box 1).

Qualitative Inquiry and the Politics of Research edited by Norman K. Denzin and Michael D. Giardina, 119–139. © 2015 Left Coast Press, Inc. All rights reserved.

Box 1: Topics of ICQI as a development

2005 Qualitative Inquiry in a Time of *Global Uncertainty*

2006 *Ethics*, Politics, and Human Subject Research

2007 Qualitative Inquiry and the *Politics of Evidence*

2008 Ethics, *Evidence*, and Social Justice

2009 Advancing *Human Rights* Through Qualitative Research

2010 Qualitative Inquiry For a *Global Community* in Crisis

2011 Qualitative Inquiry and the *Politics of Advocacy*

2012 Qualitative Inquiry as a *Global Endeavour*

2013 Qualitative Inquiry *Outside the Academy*

2014 Qualitative Inquiry and the *Politics of Research*

(taken from icqi.org; italics added)

The thematic lines across the ten years show how the congress has always tried to link qualitative inquiry to bigger issues: it has shed light on general circumstances such as global uncertainty and communities in crisis. The roles of research in general and qualitative inquiry in particular are discussed with the focus on politics of evidence and advocacy. This year's (2014) issue, the politics of research, can be seen as a general summary of these perspectives. This chapter, however, is not about the history or development of qualitative inquiry in retrospection. Rather, it wants to locate progress of qualitative inquiry in this context when it addresses current and future developments, trends, and challenges. In more detail, it will address the following issues and run through the following steps:

• Politics of research
• Societal relevance of qualitative inquiry
• A globalized view of qualitative research
• Doing qualitative research, the meanings and uses of data

- Proliferation of qualitative research
- Recovering qualitative research from current trends
- Internationalization of qualitative research
- Trends and challenges for the future

Politics of Research

In what follows, politics of research is understood as that we use our potentials of doing research for academic and societal purposes—which means to further establish qualitative inquiry and to use it for addressing societal relevant problems.

Our projects, for example those we do in Berlin, often pass through the following steps if we want to make a contribution of *societal relevance* with qualitative methods:

- Identify vulnerable groups in society
- Identify social problems these groups are confronted with
- For example the non-utilization of social services and support
- Analyze how the institutions deal with these problems
- Use (-fullness) of research
- Relevance and implementation

If we take an example of our recent research in Germany (see also Flick, 2012), this could become more concrete as follows:

- Homeless adolescents in Germany as a vulnerable group
- Health and illness problems of this group in general as the (social) problem
- Chronic illness in this context remains untreated in particular as an example of non-utilization of services and support
- Perception of the group and institutional barriers in institutions as ways of (institutional) dealing with these problems
- Make political suggestions for how to change this situation on a more general level as a way of making the research used and useful
- Make suggestions for change the service routines as steps towards relevance and implementation of the research.

Societal Relevance of Qualitative Inquiry

Seen in the perspective of the *politics of qualitative research*, this means that in this case qualitative research is addressing social problems of vulnerable groups by making a contribution. In many cases, like in this example, the power of qualitative research comes also from the fact that it is able to work with hard-to-reach groups. These groups otherwise often refuse to participate in research, or are too small to become visible in representative studies. With projects like this one, we can *increase the acceptance* of qualitative research in disciplines like medicine, health, and political sciences, or in the realms of public and political administration, or funding institutions, as this research may demonstrate the *societal relevance* of qualitative inquiry.

However, such research currently faces a number of challenges coming from different angles. Two of these challenges will be discussed here.

Challenge I: Trends to Clusters, 'Big Data,' and 'Big Research'

In the article already mentioned, Helga Novotny (2014) highlighted several trends on the level of the research politics and funding of the European Union. These trends in funding lead to advancing 'big research,' big data, interdisciplinary research (of social sciences with natural sciences), and the integration of research funding into bigger programs of political program development. For German contexts, we can currently state a trend of research funding toward *financing big clusters* (of many projects coming from several disciplines). This funding is intended not only to finance the study and answer research questions and social problems, it is also (or even more) intended to build up and change the structure of universities—by establishing clusters of excellence. In Germany, for example, the Research Council spent more than half of its 2009 budget on such clusters (Meier & Schimank, 2014). This trend has been growing—at the mercy of the number of funded projects like the above example, which had been funded by this source. In these developments, the chances for obtaining and funding for studies like the above example become smaller and smaller.

Challenge II: Applying Qualitative Research in Different Cultures

The second challenge is coming from the growing need to extend such research beyond our local cultures. In our above example, the population of homeless adolescents in Germany has become much more international in recent years with more and more members coming from Eastern Europe, for example. Continuing such research means that we increasingly have to address people migrating from one culture to the other. So we face the challenge of how to apply qualitative research methods in different cultures.

A Globalized View of Qualitative Research

This raises issues linked to the trend of globalizing qualitative research and, more particularly, linked to using qualitative research for analyzing experiences and issues of migration. We addressed this issue in panels at this congress in more detail in 2012, and a special issue in Qualitative Inquiry about this has just been published (Flick, 2014a). If we extend our research in this direction, we face challenges on five levels (see Flick & Röhnsch, 2014, p. 1105):

- Concepts of research
- Issues of access
- Doing interviews
- Analyzing the data
- Data between cultures

One of our ongoing research projects is about the utilization of institutions of drug and addiction treatment in Germany by migrants from countries of the former Soviet Union. We face these challenges in this project in more concrete terms:

- Concepts of research: Qualitative methods and participants' views
- Issues of access: Hard to reach groups and language
- Doing interviews: Working with translators/interpreters
- Analyzing the data: Interpretation between two cultures
- Data between cultures: Cultural concepts of addiction

Our understanding of research—non-directive interviews and ethnography—is not always compatible with what our migrants have experienced as research in their countries of origin and expect from social scientists. As several authors have discussed, our understanding of using interviews is in conflict with what people with a Russian background see as research—they expect clear question and answer schemes instead of open-ended questions (see, for example: Fröhlich, 2012; Weaver, 2011). Gobo (2011) has highlighted the implicit assumptions the use of interviews is based on and how these are rooted in a Western, democratic concept of society.

The second challenge is to find access to such a hard-to-reach group and to overcome the language barrier here. Sometimes, working with native speaking researchers helps to bridge the language gap. In some of our cases, however, Russian-speaking researchers were viewed with mistrust and negative associations related to a history of interrogations in their countries of origin (Flick & Röhnsch, 2014). In interviews and ethnography, it becomes necessary for qualitative researchers to work with translators and interpreters (Littig & Pöchhacker, 2014). Then we have to take into account their influence on the interview situation and on what is said. Alternatives for dealing with their roles are to try to minimize the translators' influences or to aim at making them an explicit part of the research situation (Edwards, 1998). When we want to understand the specific problems and experiences of a migrant group (e.g., Russian speaking migrants) in the German health and addiction care system, we need to reflect on how to take culture and cultures into account when analyzing the data without neglecting, but also without overemphasizing, them. Not to use available support can also be observed in drug users coming from Germany, but the aim of our research is to identify the culture specific barriers and obstacles. A particular challenge is then to reveal the cultural concepts of addiction behind our interviewees' statements and the differences to our (and the service system's) concepts.

On a methodological level, these challenges for qualitative research can be summarized in two more general questions:

• How to take this need for a culture sensitive use of qualitative research into account when applying qualitative methods in different cultures or in ethnic groups in a society with a different linguistic and cultural background?

- How to adapt methods in the process?

Doing Qualitative Research, the Meanings and Uses of Data

The first part of this chapter has mainly addressed qualitative research in some general respects and thus referred to the first keyword in its title ('qualitative'). Now it will focus on the second part of the title ('data') and on issues of 'doing qualitative research, the meanings and uses of data' (borrowing a phrase from the Director's welcome to this Congress—Denzin, 2014). On the background of editing the *SAGE Handbook of Qualitative Data Analysis* (Flick, 2014b), the following issues have become significant:

- Using existing/natural occurring data or elicited data;
- Data analysis as applying methods (e.g., Grounded Theory coding) to whatever sort of data (interviews, observation, etc.);
- Data analysis as approaches specifically developed for the type of data to be analyzed (interviews, observation, virtual data);
- Triangulation of both approaches.

Uses of Data in the Analysis

Qualitative research has always oscillated between using two kinds of data: (1) in conversation analysis of mundane conversations, *natural or existing* data are the basis of research. Other approaches are based (2) on *producing or eliciting new* data in interviews or ethnography, for example.

When it comes to analyzing data, we can see two major approaches: One is to take *existing methods*—such as Grounded Theory coding (Thornberg & Charmaz, 2014)—and to *apply* them to the concrete data (interviews, observation, etc.) in the project. The alternative is to *take the type of data as a starting point* and to use approaches specifically *developed for analyzing* interviews (see Roulston, 2014, for example)—this means to start the other way round. Finally, for both distinctions, we can consider *triangulating* both approaches by using existing data (e.g., documents) and combining them with elicited data (e.g., interviews). In a similar way we can combine approaches specific for analyzing documents (see Coffey, 2014) with applying Grounded Theory coding for example.

These distinctions lead to another issue, which is quite important for the points that will be addressed later. If we look back on the development of qualitative research, we see the proliferation of qualitative research into a number of schools of research. Prominent schools in qualitative research (see Flick, 2014c, ch. 31) are

- Grounded theory;
- Ethnomethodology and conversation analysis;
- Discourse analysis;
- Narrative analysis and biographical research;
- Phenomenology;
- Ethnography and auto-ethnography;
- Performance oriented research;
- Action research.

Schools tend to become autonomous from a more general discussion in the discipline, to develop their own research traditions and fields, distinctive kinds of research questions, methods, and so forth. At the same time, if the general landscapes of social sciences or qualitative research are changing, single schools may be affected more strongly by such changes or get along better with them than others.

In the next step a number of current trends qualitative research is currently confronted with or undergoing will be addressed as examples for changing landscapes. Given the variety in qualitative research, it is not sure whether the following trends will lead to progress for each of these approaches or whether they might lead to losing some of these schools along the way.

Recovering Qualitative Research from Current Trends

In the current international landscape of qualitative research the following trends can be identified as *relevant but not unproblematic* for our current state of affairs:

- Qualitative research in the archives: Research infrastructures;
- Re-use and re-analysis of qualitative data;
- Ethics and serendipity;
- Discovery of qualitative research in the context of evidence;
- Triangulation in the context of mixed methods.

Research Infrastructures in and for Qualitative Research

The first trend is based on the expectation that qualitative data should not only be produced for the concrete research project they are created for but should also be made available for a wider public of researchers or other audiences. In Germany again, we find a pressure in funding institutions and research politicians and managers to build up 'research infra-structures.' Arguments mentioned for such a development are, first, that research infrastructures are a precondition for societal relevance of social and qualitative research:

> Research infra-structures make a substantial contribution in all scientific areas to the scientific production of knowledge to the scientific answering of questions of societal relevance and to the international links of such efforts. (Wissenschaftsrat, 2011, p. 7)

A second argument refers to the quality of research seen as depending on the establishment of archiving and availability of qualitative data for other researchers:

> As a replication of studies in the realm of qualitative research ... normally is not possible, the inter-subjective transparency of scientific statements on the basis of the existing primary data is a major quality criterion of qualitative research. Losing such data is particularly sensitive against this background. (Wissenschaftsrat, 2011, pp. 56–57)

These statements show that the claim in this development is not only to make available results but also to make available the primary data and the coding instruments or intermediary findings.

Archiving Qualitative Research as a New Standard?

The idea of developing such infra-structures is often linked to the idea of building up archives where data are stored, available, and accessible for other researchers and studies. Archiving qualitative research raises a number of questions.

Archiving in Qualitative Research: Open Questions

The first set of these questions refers to the role of context in qualitative research and how far archiving bears the danger of decontextualizing data and research: Can we use and re-use qualitative data in a meaningful way without really knowing the context of data collection and the methodological particularities and taking them into account? To do qualitative data analysis without being involved in the context of research, without referring to the original research questions pursued with them or which they were produced for may lead to rather bloodless and abstract findings. To produce such decontextualized data is not really what qualitative research is about. The aim and claim of archiving as a standard and building up infra-structures for qualitative research, to allow other researchers to take the data out of their original context and to assess and re-use them widely, may have some appeal. But the challenge is how to really take into account the contexts in the data, which is an essential part of the narrative interview, for example, in furthering or re-using data in secondary analyses. In particular, when data (e.g., statements) are embedded in a more extensive structure, such as a narrative or ethnography, it will be difficult to re-use them without seeing this context as essential. This leads to the *major question* here: Which kinds of data of research of approaches/schools fit into archives and the expectations linked to them?

This trend is not only embedded in making qualitative data available for other researchers but also to make them available for other kinds of research, such as meta-analysis. The second trend here is to re-use and re-analyze qualitative data and to expect that qualitative research will be able to provide this.

Re-using Qualitative Data: Qualitative Meta-analysis

This trend also extends the argumentation to the third part of the title of this chapter—trends in data *analysis*. Several strategies for qualitative meta-analysis have been discussed now for some time (see Timulak, 2014):

- Meta-study (Paterson et al., 2001)
  - –meta-data-analysis;
  - –meta-method;
  - –meta-theory.
- Metasummary (Sandelowski & Barroso, 2007)
  - –extraction of findings from primary studies;
  - –abstraction of those findings; and
  - –calculation of effect sizes.

To go into detail about how the concrete approaches work is beyond this chapter. But two more general remarks seem necessary. First, our discussion does not mean that it is per se a bad idea to import the approach of meta-analysis into the realm of qualitative research. The more results can unfold a bigger contribution to answering relevant questions in this way, the better it is. However, again, if such an approach becomes a *general* trend or even a general expectation—qualitative data and research have to be ready for re-analysis—the danger is that a lot of the variety of doing qualitative research and of the data we produce will not fit in such re-analysis schemes. For example, statements from interviews will fit in such schemes much easier than descriptions coming from observation protocols in ethnography. If availability and readiness for re-analysis become pre-conditions for funding or for integrating approaches in teaching, the danger again is that we lose parts of the variety and the openness of qualitative research. The challenges here are:

- How far does the trend to meta-analysis, metasynthesis, and so forth lead to new implicit or explicit standards for qualitative research (at least if to consider)?

• Will this reduce the openness and variety in qualitative research?

The third trend here has again to do with an issue that is very important and in general a must in the discussion of qualitative research.

Ethics and Serendipity

Research ethics, informed consent, and a review by an ethics committee are important contributions to making research better and improving researchers' responsibility for their participants. Following the issues just discussed, the following practical and at the same time more general problem becomes relevant: If we start interviews, for example, by asking participants for their (informed) consent, are such permissions for doing research or the informed consents obtained valid for re-use of data for all purposes and for every other researcher? What does this mean for clearances by ethic committees? We should reflect how far in every case a general permit for collecting data and using them in the current project and using them in any kind of later project is desirable. This means the trend to making qualitative data widely available also independently from the context for which they are originally collected produces a number of ethical issues and consequences. This can make the actual research much more complicated and questionable.

Working in fields like the above examples from our research has raised another question: What does it mean if we have obtained beforehand the ethical permissions for interviewing specific people (e.g., patients) and find out in running our study that we need other interviewees or other methods for answering our research questions? Such extensions and shifts are not uncommon in a flexible research strategy such as ethnography or exploratory research projects. With Robert Merton this approach to research can also be labeled as 'serendipity' (Merton & Barber, 2004). How far does the (necessary) ethical grounding of our research delimit the flexibility of our research practice in this sense—as an essential of qualitative research different from standardized quantitative research—in an inappropriate way? How do we deal with this?

Discovery of Qualitative Research in the Context of Evidence-based Politics

If we come back now to the more general topics of infrastructure, archiving, and meta-analysis or re-analysis, these trends can be seen in the context of another big issue which has quite intensely puzzled ICQI congresses in earlier years. At that time a specific danger was seen and discussed as the predominant issue—that qualitative research will be pushed away or run over by the "elephant in the living room" to borrow again an illustrative phrase by Norman Denzin (2009). Currently, another trend and danger should be noticed. In several areas in health research, for example, the classical model of evidence finds its limits. A way out of this kind of dead end is to rediscover qualitative research for this context.

In more recent publications of the Cochrane Institute (in evidence-based intervention oriented health research) we read about a new interest in qualitative research:

Currently, there are four possibilities to make use of qualitative research in the context of Cochrane Intervention reviews:

- The use of qualitative research to define and refine review questions (informing reviews).

- The use of qualitative research identified while looking for evidence of effectiveness (enhancing reviews).

- The use of findings derived from a specific search for qualitative evidence that addresses questions related to an effectiveness review (extending reviews).

- Conducting a qualitative evidence synthesis to address questions other than effectiveness (supplementing reviews) (Hannes, 2011, p. 2).

In this discussion our earlier point about re-analysis and meta-analysis becomes relevant again in a specific way—by producing reports based on synthesizing evidence from qualitative research. This is spelled out in more concrete terms:

Qualitative evidence synthesis is a process of combining evidence from individual qualitative studies to create new understanding by comparing and analyzing concepts and findings from different sources of evidence with a focus on the same topic of interest.

Therefore, qualitative evidence synthesis can be considered a complete study in itself, comparable to any meta-analysis within a systematic review on effects of interventions or diagnostic tests. (Higgins & Green, 2011, ch. 20.3.2.3)

Again, this can be seen as a trend with positive sides to it—more recognition of qualitative research and results and at the same time maybe more impact of our research as outlined at the beginning of this chapter. However, this comes again with a number of challenges. If such recognition of qualitative research is seen as desirable, the question arises, how far new standards and claims of quality are defined for qualitative research through the backdoor. Furthermore, this may have a more general consequence, if it leads to a limited understanding of what is accepted as acceptable qualitative research.

The last trend to mention here brings us back to qualitative research in general. This trend has been taken up with some enthusiasm, sometimes critically (sometimes even featured in an extra day of sessions), and is part of the current program of ICQI again.

Triangulation in the Context of Mixed Methods

Initially inaugurated by Denzin (1970), the idea of "triangulation," that is, using more than one method or, more generally, more than one approach in our research, has been quite prominent in qualitative research. We can refer here to the ups and downs of 'triangulation' as a concept. The downs have at some points been intensified by turning to 'mixed methods' as a new concept coming with a lot of extra claims—from being the better concept, to being less limited than triangulation, to being the answer to the paradigm wars and to being the solution to the juxtaposition of qualitative and quantitative research in general. Again, we should appreciate that this can be a fruitful approach for some issues of research, but mention one caveat: If we look at the mission statement of the *Journal of Mixed Methods Research* (JMMR), we find a clear focus:

Mixed methods research is defined as research in which the investigator collects and analyzes data, integrates the findings, and draws inferences using both qualitative and quantitative approaches or methods in a single study or program of inquiry. (JMMR Mission Statement)

But in the research examples mentioned before it may have become obvious already that we need more than one approach in such studies. We need here a systematic triangulation of perspectives (Flick, 1992) in the encounter of vulnerable groups and service providers. We do not need quantitative methods, but we need to do *interviews* with the members of the vulnerable groups about their expectations towards services and help, and their expectations in regard to trying to find help or why they refrain from utilizing the services. We also need *expert interviews* with the service providers' staff in order to their view on this clientele and their view on existing barriers against utilization of professional help. Finally, we need an *ethnographic approach* for understanding the practices of both sides. With a systematic triangulation of perspectives we can understand the process of "doing social problems" in this field (see Figure 5.1).

Of course, this is not a general model of doing qualitative research, but this example should illustrate that we need a broader understanding of working with multiple methods beyond what is understood as mixed methods (see also Flick et al., 2012, for the possible relations of triangulation and mixed methods).

Figure 5.1: Triangulation of perspectives in the study of doing social problems

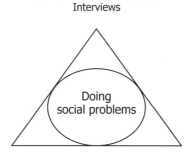

Clients' views and attitudes:
Interviews

Doing
social problems

Institution and administration
as barriers: Expert interviews

Circumstances; Clients as victims
of their situations: Ethnography

Internationalizing Qualitative Research

Earlier, this chapter addressed the use of qualitative research in the context of globalization of issues and of the range of participants we work with. Extending this issue, a more general discussion refers to the question of how we can promote more strongly a development towards an internationalization of qualitative research. This need has been spelled out from various angles. Ping-Chun Hsiung (2012), for example, has problematized a core-periphery divide between local traditions and cultures of research in Asia (periphery) and the mainstream discussions and textbooks in the Anglo-American (core) area of qualitative research. The main issue here is how far offers from core discussion are appropriate for what the periphery needs. More concretely, the mainstream discussions appear to be imported at the cost of the local traditions, maybe pushing them aside. Finally, mainstream textbooks and examples are seen as less helpful for teaching in other cultural contexts. Alasuutari (2004) had suggested reconsidering the history of qualitative research by using a spatial approach emphasizing local traditions of qualitative research rather than stressing a timeline of methodological progress (as in earlier editions of the Handbook of Denzin & Lincoln, 2011, for example). The situation of qualitative research in Germany may illustrate the need for such a spatial approach. Here, distinct approaches to qualitative research have been quite prominent in the research and methodological discussions in the last four decades. Examples are the 'Narrative Interview,' developed in the early 1970s (see Rosenthal, 2004), and the 'Objective Hermeneutics,' developed in the 1970s (see Wernet, 2014). These approaches have hardly been recognized in international discussions, for example, at the ICQI congresses, in Anglo-Saxon journals, handbooks, and textbooks. The same might be the case for other local developments in countries like France, Italy, or in Eastern Europe, Asia, and so forth (see also Flick, 2014d, and Knoblauch, Flick & Maeder, 2005). These brief remarks may illustrate that there is still a lot to do for establishing a really internationalized or globalized development of qualitative research.

Trends and Challenges for the Future of Qualitative Research

Rounding up what has been said so far, the following questions are still waiting for satisfying answers:

- How to make qualitative research really international, global, and local.
- How to make qualitative research really societally relevant without boiling it down to limited variations (just interviews, just results).
- How to adapt it to new contexts (e.g., citizen research), uses, and phenomena (data).

Looking into the future and daring to set a prognosis for the critical cutting edge of 20 years—where will we be after 20 years of ICQI? Here we can see two possible perspectives. The first could be outlined as: "Maybe they don't need us anymore." Nigel Fielding (2014, p. 1066) describes a current major trend:

> The rise of 'citizen research' via online media is likely to entail unpredictable changes in the practice and purposes of social research because we would have to go back to the invention of the printing press for a socio-technological development of equivalent magnitude.

In particular, approaches such as 'extreme citizen science' will maybe enable and empower broader audiences and everyday people to take our methods and do their own research with them. Thus, they will maybe abandon the idea of the experts of research—as methodologists, as researchers, as scientists.

> Extreme Citizen Science is a situated, bottom-up practice that takes into account local needs, practices and culture and works with broad networks of people to design and build new devices and knowledge creation processes that can transform the world. (EXTREME CITIZEN SCIENCE (EXCITES) UCL London www.ucl.ac.uk/excites)

The second possible perspective could be: Maybe it's just us? For example, a recent editorial of the journal, *Work, Employment and Society,* has stated:

> According to the recent benchmarking review of the discipline, UK sociological research is predominantly based around qualitative research methods …. Further, evidence suggests that the overwhelming majority of empirical articles published in mainstream UK sociology journals are qualitative in their focus. (Charlwood et al., 2014, p. 155)

This means that in some contexts, qualitative research will take over certain disciplines, the research, the teaching, the publications and so on—maybe not the worst outcome of a long struggle for establishing qualitative research as a major element in social and other sciences.

Conclusion

Coming back to the title of this chapter, what does 'qualitative data analysis 2.0' mean here? It means to develop, adapt, and pursue qualitative research along the following lines:

- To take on the chances and challenges of the trends discussed in this chapter;
- To take care that the impact on qualitative inquiry is non-reductionist and to keep it alive;
- To adapt qualitative research, data, and analysis to the new global and local needs;
- To try to stay relevant in changing circumstances;
- To keep on reflecting but also doing qualitative research; and more generally:
- To keep on keeping on!

References

Alasuutari, P. (2004). The globalization of qualitative research. In C. Seale, G. Gobo, J. F. Gubrium & D. Silverman (Eds.), *Qualitative research practice* (pp. 595–608). London: Sage.

Charlwood, A., Forde, C., Grugulis I., Hardy, K., Kirkpatrick, I., MacKenzie, R., & Stuart, M. (2014). Clear, rigorous and relevant: Publishing quantitative research articles in *Work, employment and society. Work, Employment and Society*, 2014, *28*(2), 155–167.

Coffey, A. (2014). Analyzing documents. In U. Flick (Ed.), *The SAGE handbook of qualitative data analysis* (pp. 367–379). London: Sage.

Denzin, N. K. (1970). *The research act.* Englewood Cliffs, NJ: Prentice Hall.

Denzin, N. K (2009). The elephant in the living room: Or extending the conversation about the politics of evidence. *Qualitative Research*, *9*(2), 139–160.

Denzin, N. K. (2014). Welcome from the director. *ICQI Program 2014* (p. 14). Available from www.ICQI.org

Denzin, N. K., & Lincoln, Y. S. (Eds.) (2011). *The SAGE handbook of qualitative research* (4th ed.). London: Sage.

Edwards, R. (1998). A critical examination of the use of interpreters in the qualitative research process. *Journal of Ethnic and Migration Studies*, *24*, 197–208.

Fielding, N. G. (2014). Qualitative research and our digital futures. *Qualitative Inquiry*, *20*, 9, 1064–1073.

Flick, U. (1992). Triangulation revisited: Strategy of or alternative to validation of qualitative data. *Journal for the Theory of Social Behavior*, *22*, 175–197.

Flick, U. (2012). Vulnerability and the politics of advocacy: Challenges for qualitative inquiry using multiple methods. In N. Denzin & M. Giardina (Eds.), *Qualitative inquiry and the politics of advocacy* (pp. 163–182). Walnut Creek, CA: Left Coast Press, Inc.

Flick, U. (Ed.). (2014a). Special issue 'Qualitative research as global endeavor.' *Qualitative Inquiry, 20* (9).

Flick, U. (Ed.). (2014b). *The SAGE handbook of qualitative data analysis.* London: Sage.

Flick, U. (2014c). *An introduction to qualitative research* (5th ed.). London: Sage.

Flick, U. (2014d). Challenges for qualitative inquiry as a global endeavor—Introduction to the special issue. *Qualitative Inquiry*, *20*(9), 1059–1063.

Flick, U., & Röhnsch, R. (2014). Migrating diseases—Triangulating approaches: Applying qualitative inquiry as a global endeavor. *Qualitative Inquiry*, *20*(9), 1096–1109.

Flick, U., Garms-Homolová, V., Herrmann, W. J., Kuck, J., & Röhnsch, G. (2012). 'I can't prescribe something just because someone asks for it …': Using mixed methods in the framework of triangulation. *Journal of Mixed Methods Research, 6*(2), 97–110.

Fröhlich, C. (2012). Interviewforschung im russisch-sprachigen Raum— ein Balanceakt zwischen methodologischen und feldspezifischen Ansprüchen [Interview research in the Russian-speaking area—An act balancing between methodological and field specific demands]. In J. Kruse, S. Bethmann, D. Niemann & C. Schmieder (Eds.), *Qualitative Interviewforschung in und mit fremden Sprachen* (pp. 186–202). Weinheim, Germany: Beltz Juventa.

Gobo, G. (2011). Globalizing methodology? The encounter between local methodologies. *International Journal of Social Research Methodology, 14*, 417–437.

Hannes, K. (2011). Chapter 4: Critical appraisal of qualitative research. In J. Noyes, A. Booth, K. Hannes, A. Harden, J. Harris, S. Lewin & C. Lockwood (Eds.), *Supplementary guidance for inclusion of qualitative research in Cochrane systematic reviews of interventions.* Version 1 (updated August 2011). Cochrane Collaboration Qualitative Methods Group, 2011. Available from cqrmg.cochrane.org/supplemental-handbook-guidance

Higgins, J. P. T., & Green, S. (Eds.) (2011). *Cochrane handbook for systematic reviews of interventions.* Available from handbook.cochrane.org

Hsiung, P.-C. (2012). The globalization of qualitative research: Challenging Anglo-American domination and local hegemonic discourse. *Forum Qualitative Sozialforschung/Forum: Qualitative Social Research, 13*(1), Article 21. Retrieved from nbn-resolving.de/urn:nbn:de:0114-fqs1201216

Knoblauch, H., Flick, U., & Maeder, C. (Eds.). (2005). The state of the art of qualitative research in Europe [Special issue]. *Forum Qualitative Sozialforschung/Forum: Qualitative Social Research, 6*(3). Retrieved from www.qualita- tive-research.net/fqs/fqs-e/inhalt3-05-e.htm

Littig, B., & Pöchhacker, F. (2014). Socio-translational collaboration in qualitative inquiry: The case of expert interviews. *Qualitative Inquiry, 20*(9), 1085–1095.

Meier, F., & Schimank, U. (2014). Cluster-building and the transformation of the university. *Soziologie, 43*(2), 139–166.

Merton, R. K., & Barber, E. (2004). *The travels and adventures of serendipity: A study in sociological semantics and the sociology of science.* Princeton, NJ: Princeton University Press.

Novotny, H. (2014). Ein gemeinnütziges Labor für die Gesellschaft. In HIS (Ed.), *50 Jahre HIS—Festschrift* (pp. 16–21). Vienna: HIS.

Paterson, B. L., Thorne, S. E., Canam, C., & Jillings, C. (2001). *Meta-study of qualitative health research: A practical guide to meta-analysis and meta-synthesis.* Thousand Oaks, CA: Sage.

Rosenthal, G. (2004). Biographical research. In C. Seale, G. Gobo, J. Gubrium & D. Silverman (Eds.), *Qualitative research practice* (pp. 48–65). London: Sage.

Roulston, K. (2014). Analyzing interviews. In U. Flick (Ed.), *The SAGE handbook of qualitative data analysis* (pp. 297–312). London: Sage.

Sandelowski, M., & Barroso, J. (Eds.). (2007). *Handbook for synthesizing qualitative research.* New York: Springer.

Thornberg, R., & Charmaz, K. (2014). Grounded theory and theoretical coding. In U. Flick (Ed.), *The SAGE handbook of qualitative data analysis* (pp. 153–169). London: Sage.

Timulak, L. (2014). Qualitative meta-analysis. In U. Flick (Ed.), *The SAGE handbook of qualitative data analysis* (pp. 481–495). London: Sage.

Weaver, D. (2011). Neither too scientific nor a spy: Negotiating the ethnographic interview in Russia. *Comparative Sociology, 10,* 145–157.

Wernet, A. (2014). Hermeneutics and objective hermeneutics. In U. Flick (Ed.), *The SAGE handbook of qualitative data analysis* (pp. 234–246). London: Sage.

Wissenschaftsrat. (2011). *Empfehlungen zu Forschungsinfrastrukturen in den Geistes- und Sozialwissenschaften.* Available at www. wissenschaftsrat.de/download/archiv/10465-11.pdf [04.04.2013]

Chapter 6

Critical Autoethnography as Intersectional Praxis

A Performative Pedagogical Interplay on Bleeding Borders of Identity[1]

Bryant Keith Alexander

For me, doing critical autoethnography is sometimes like capturing a picture of yourself in a glass, borderless frame; a picture in which an image of you is represented and there are sightless borders of containment; containments called race, sex, gender, culture, and occasions of human social experience fixed in time and space, floating in a fixed liquidity of memory, giving shape to experience, structuring vision and engagement with the intent for others to see and know you differently as you story the meaningfulness of personal experience in a cultural context. For me, this is the engagement of autoethnography. The critical in critical autoethnography captures a moment in that borderless frame and holds it to a particular scrutiny—intersplicing a sociology-of-the-self with a hermeneutics of theorizing the self. Yet, in the process of such an engagement, there is always a feeling of risk: a risk of bleeding, in which the presumed categorical containments of your identity threaten to exceed its borders, revealing the ways in which we are always both particular and plural at the same time; never contained and always messy.

From Boylorn, Robin M. and Mark P. Orbe. 2013. *Critical Autoethnography: Intersecting Cultural Identities in Everyday Life.* © Left Coast Press, Inc. Republished in *Qualitative Inquiry and the Politics of Research* edited by Norman K. Denzin and Michael D. Giardina, 141–157. (Left Coast Press, Inc., 2015). All rights reserved.

I often have used the construct of "bleeding borders" or "bleeding identities" to reference the false boundaries that limit social possibility—whether that be the migration of identities across place and space, or the limitations of what we are supposed to be, based on the materiality of bodies, the presumed fixity of sex and gender, or the historical points of origin that signal cultural and clan affiliation (see, for example, Alexander, 2011). I have argued that the notion of "bleeding" is not necessarily a violent metaphor, as much as the travel between permeable membranes of bordered identities within an embodied text—often when inter/intra-cultural-racial encounters force a realization of the predicament of selves. Such a construction in my engagement of a critical autoethnography also reveals the intersectional nature of identity.

In her oft-cited essay, "Mapping the Margins: Intersectionality, Identity Politics, and Violence against Women," Kimberlé Crenshaw (1995) offers the construct of *intersectionality*, which examines the intersection of race (particularly African American raced identity) with gender (particularly African American women). In her conclusions, she speaks to

> recognizing that identity politics takes place at the site where categories intersect thus seems more fruitful than challenging the possibility of talking about categories at all. Through an awareness of intersectionality, we can better acknowledge and ground the differences among us and negotiate the means by which these differences will find expression in constructing group politics. (p. 377)

For me, in doing critical autoethnography you always experience odd moments of catching a glimpse of yourself in a glass, borderless frame; images of yourself reflecting back from the gloss and glean of a polished surface layered atop the fixed image *of* yourself, a potentially reified rendition caught in time; a ghosting, if you will, that when viewed, forces a critical reflexive moment of searching for the missing pieces of yourself that the shutter of the lens did not capture but only critical autoethnography can recover—revealing the dynamic of politics at play in the scene that at once appears fixed but in actuality bleeds the lives narrated in the picture and the very moment of viewing the picture itself. So, it is in this way that I want to begin this exploration of critical autoethnography as intersectional praxis, and as a particular pedagogy of doing.

Trying to Tell the Story of a Borderless Frame

There is a story that I want to tell. No, there is a story that I *need* to tell. A story claimed by others that will be told, whether I like it or not, but it won't include my voice. It won't include my side. It won't include me in the manner that I want to be re/presented. It won't include me trying to make sense of the story in the process of thinking and writing the story. It won't include the story of me stepping back to see the story with perspective; the story of me stepping back from the picture to see me in the picture of the story trying to get perspective; the story of me stepping back to critically see me and others in the story I tell, knowing that it is not exclusively my story (nor theirs). In this moment I am not staging a moment that reifies a given reality, but taking stock of how I am implicated in the scene of a happening. Maybe I will be "read" in this story. Maybe the story is really in that photo. That photo that sits on the shelf in my living room that everyone makes comments about. That photo of my three brothers and me, the one from the wedding:

> His wedding, and
>
> His wedding, and
>
> His wedding, but not my wedding.
>
> That photo.

That *queer* photo of three straight Black men dressed in white tuxedoes and one queer Black man dressed in a tan suit. Me, still with long hair that they joke makes me look feminine, in relation to their own performed masculinity in which the length of hair becomes a politic of gender. It's not a joke, it is a critique and one that in my childhood far preceded the dreadlocks that later grew as an act of resistance from my head.

> Brothers.
>
> Brothers?

That photo that *I* staged and had someone take. That photo that *I* gave a copy of to each of them, pressed behind a prism of glass with a borderless frame, implicates me. It implicates them. A borderless frame, as if there are no limits to its containment or limits to the interpretations by which every brother tells a story.

It is a wedding photo.

It is a photo taken at a wedding.

It is a photo of my three brothers and me.

It is a photo that weds us to each/other.

It is a wedding photo that I am allowed to be in but I can't be part of the wedding.

Each of the brothers in white is married. Each of the brothers in white invited the other brothers to be in their wedding. I received no such invitations. This picture is performativity; the iteration of an iteration, of an iteration, maybe of an intention. But that's my story. The story that I gave them in a borderless frame. In the picture I am the anomaly. I am the irregularity. I am the peculiarity. I am the queer. Invited to attend the wedding, but not to be in the wedding. Not invited to wed. That photo of my three brothers and me, the one from the wedding; from the symbolic weddings:

His wedding, and

His wedding, and

His wedding, but not my wedding.

Invited to attend the weddings, but not to be in the weddings.

Not invited to wed.

I staged this photo as I am staging this story to document our brotherhood, not realizing that the abject body in the photo (and maybe in the story) would be mine. The queer brother in tan also standing in place for the absent queer brother, a fifth brother, who died from AIDS before the weddings; another tan suit? We called him Tanny, which was short for Nathanial. I am implicated in the staging of this photo. I am implicated in the telling of this story. I am implicated in this story through a complicity of blood, gender, race, and writing. This story is not apolitical.

It is a story about brothers and gender performance.

It is a story about the heterosexual privilege to wed.

It is a story about inclusion, exclusion, and bordered and borderless identities that bleed in the banal moments of weddings, and photos, and the mixed identities of brothers (biological, cultural, racial, or spiritual). It is a story about the intersectionality of identity; a meeting place of race, sexuality, culture, and gender; co-informing, co-narrating and co-performing identities that become something altogether different, more. I don't know their stories.

It is a picture that I love.

It is a picture that I hate.

It is a picture that I hate to love.

It is a picture that I study with critical intent to find my selves floating in a fixed liquidity of identity politics.

In the presence of my brothers I am the same and not the same. I am a Black man linked with other black men by biology and heritage. Yet the particularity of sexuality, their heterosexuality and my homosexuality, becomes the perceptual variable that marks our difference—in that way in which our relational dynamic is both intraracial and intercultural at the same time.

▪

In using autoethnography as a critical methodology in performance studies classes and even classes like interpersonal, relational, and intercultural communication, I have often asked students to engage in an explication of lived experience in a cultural context; exploring themselves in relation to and in the context of cultural communities. But in particular, I have asked them to do a performed close analysis of their identity as a critical nexus. Following Crenshaw (1995), I am asking students to not easily settle on the particularity of their race, sex, and gender or even the more amorphous constructions of culture and class in which they glom onto a collective sense of self as practiced in alignment with others. I ask them to address the bleeding borders of their identity that place them betwixt and between; places and times in which the seeming singularity of their identity becomes plural. In an autoethnographic assignment, I ask them to speak to variables of personality, positionality, and the politics of being that dynamize their sense of self in relation to culture and society.

Hence, Crenshaw's construction of intersectionality is helpful as an analytical tool in teaching this approach to autoethnography without the limitation of only focusing on race, sex, and gender. In some ways, maybe I am engaging what Wenshu Lee (2012) references as a *critical intersectionality* that expands the "holy trinity of identity markers, race, class and gender" to such variables as "age, religiosity, ideology, and party identification" and more (p. 922). And while Lee does not cite Crenshaw, the intentionality of her reference is implied. And while Lee does not offer a particular definition of *the critical* in her construction of *critical intersectionality*—such a meaningful definition is at the core of my own orientation (in this approach) to teaching autoethnography and the evidenced student enactments as response to this assignment that I include in this essay.

The notion of "critical" is an engagement of discernment of the deep meanings in any given situation with the potentials and possibilities of transformation. In approaching a critical autoethnography, I often use D. Soyini Madison's orientation to doing critical work. In her construction, Madison (2005) writes that critical work seeks

> to articulate and identify hidden forces and ambiguities that operate beneath appearances; to guide judgments and evaluations emanating from our discontent; to direct our attention to the critical expressions within different interpretive communities relative to their unique symbol systems, customs, and codes; to demystify the ubiquity and magnitude of power; to provide insight and inspire acts of justice; and to name and analyze what is intuitively felt. (p. 13)

Madison's construction is aptly applied to engaging a critical autoethnography, because it asks deep questions and demands rigorous considerations. In teaching critical autoethnography, I often frame each of her definitional components as questions that students must ask themselves, thus forestalling the tendency to simply tell a good story, but to tell a critical story of meaning situated in a cultural context with potential to transform self and society (Spry, 2011). So with this framing of a critical autoethnography as intersectional praxis, I want to share with you samples of student work in a junior-level performance studies class at California State University, Los Angeles. I present two pieces with the students' permission. Each of the student efforts follows a form that might be described as a *poetic autoethnography*, both in the form of engagement as well as in that way in which poetry is a liquidity of emotion that fuses the politics of story and form.

"Advocate of Hope " by José "Pepper" Jimenez Quiroz

I was brought to a land where I had no identity, got my ID for about
a dollar 20,
so technically I was conceived at the corner store,
I never gave a damn before,
so why start now,
look into my past,
see I was born,
as an outkast,
everything I do is so unconventional,
I miss a lot of church so the music is my confessional,
it's a shame I focus on me try to make the right move,
in a year or two u gonna see me on the breaking news,
either talking recklessly,
probably making history,
doesn't really matter,
my pops facing repo,
I connect to the people standing at home depot, just like prostitutes,
tryin a get a buck or two,
tryin a get a meal,
I was born a dirty immigrant I learned to work the field,
I aint no sergeant but yea I know the drill.
My life is like a movie I just wanna see the reel.
They label me an alien,
I'm just tryin a phone home,
Look where I went wrong,
Look at my mistake,
Born in the wrong place.
Aint that a shame, my whole damn life's like Obama's campaign,
Advocate for hope, hoping for some change.

Bring it back to suspense this is just like the show,
black swan flow,
got the academy owned,
my globe aint gold,
and oscar owes more than he could afford, that's just how it goes,
stress does linger,
smiles do vanish,
every hustler on the corner first language is Spanish.
I don't smile at cops,
I hardly laugh at all,
racism hurts,
but I just laugh it off.
I been numbed by the world,
real life vicodin,
fell on the 3rd,
got right back up again.
I gotta play my cards,
there is no fold,
no bluffing when the truth is exposed,
so here I go as I testify, on my every day life, looking at me like your
life's like mine,
but you're judging from the outside, look inside of mine.
They label me an alien, I'm just tryin a phone home,
Look where I went wrong,
Look at my mistake,
Born in the wrong place,
Aint that a shame, my whole damn life's like Obama's campaign,
Advocate for hope, hoping for some change.
People where I come from usually become crooks,
they don't even see success they're scared to look.
I know about the immigrants,
didn't need to read a book,
at the age of 16 that's when my whole world shook
every moment past that, man I fully understand all the obstacles in
my path,
so I rarely show pity,
I'm labeled as a stranger in my own damn city, treating government
like my God,

I hope he forgives me.
I swear this right here is torture, me I'm the reason for the fence along
the border,
Mexican champ but I aint talking cainvalasquez,
anybody touching me on the mic, nonsense.
Mexican in the blood I can name some cartels, but me I will never
never ever tell,
not an ounce of a snitch,
I'm tryin a get big,
literally like opera.
I'm rocky balboa when it comes to tasting victory,
sorta like cesar chavez yea I'm making history.
I was born with this burden it's my original sin, green card or not I
gotta win, life's
like that, gotta face facts, I put actions in my dreams, now that's my
dream act.

■

"We Will Beat Discrimination" by Daisy Evelyn Muñiz

So something happened at 18, as I got ready for college,
It messed with my head, couldn't explain it with my own knowledge,
You see, border patrol planned raids all over my small town.
For about a month, they targeted anyone they saw was brown,
Pulling people over, even those walking the streets.
In Lake Elsinore there was a border patrol fleet
Never had I seen the town look so deserted, no one walking out their
doors,
And the thought of this, man, it shook me to my core
Man, I was scared and I was born in this nation.
But, my parents weren't, yeah, I'm the first generation
La migra took friends, co-workers, and neighbors
Good people I knew, who only wanted labor.
And I thought
We can make it through with the help of God and with
determination.
Even with the odds against us, we will beat discrimination (2x)

I closed my eyes and opened them every morn' at 3am
Wondering who else is having to do the shit I am.
Hugged and kiss my dad, we each got in our car.
Then I'd drive behind him, looked up, and wished upon a star
Daddy's little girl was now protecting him.
But, I didn't mind, yeah, I'd do it all again.
When we had driven out of town, Daddy would pull up to my side,
Turned on the light so I could see him, smiling, he'd wave bye-bye.
I'd turn mine on, wave back and smile,
releasing all the stress I'd gained with every single mile.
If I didn't do this, they might pull him over, taken him there and then
just as they had done with many other men.
As I drove home, I'd pray: God get him home safe and sound
And wondered what would happen when I moved, when I wouldn't
be around.
Oh, and I didn't mention my mom, who was basically on house arrest
'cause going out risked getting deported, just like all the rest
So that left me to take and pick up the kids, to go buy all the groceries.
Inside the stores were catholic women, whispering, holding rosaries.
I'm not catholic but I'm sure our prayers were much the same,
Lord keep us safe, we beg this in Jesus' name.
I wanted to tell them,
We can make it through with the help of God, and with
determination
Even with the odds against us, we can beat discrimination (2x)
When BP drove behind me, my heart would sink.
When I got home, I would just lay there and think,
How the hell can I be proud to be American like this
I felt so illegal, though an American miss.
I was so ashamed of being from the USA,
And I felt horrible for feeling this way.
But, it's hard when you're living like a pigeon while you're dreaming
like an eagle,
Because there's no good jobs if you are an illegal.
Things were getting outta hand, something had to be done.
So, a group of us decided to march under the IE sun.
We needed to show ICE we wouldn't take this lying down.
So, with picket signs and loud voices we marched throughout the town.

Town hall, the mayor couldn't even show his face,
All we wanted was for him to put himself in our place.
Sheriff's department, a deputy came out,
Said "sorry, this is something we can do nothing about."
The rage grew inside me; I wanted to defend my kind.
Let this border patrol pull me over, I'll give him a piece of my mind.
It frustrated me that you can stand up and be proud of that red,
white, and blue,
But, if you're not the right color, it might not be so proud of you.
Watched the news, every Spanish channel addressed the issue at least a
bit each day.
But, flip the channel to English news, and not a damn station had a
thing to say.
Did they not know, or did they simply not care.
Promoting the American dream, but they're not even playing fair.
My parents left it all for a better opportunity.
So, someone tell me why we've been suffering an eternity.
It was for me and my siblings that they stayed even when the going
got tough.
Persecuted like criminals, never once heard them say "enough is enough."
How had they endured this for so long, after 2, 3 weeks I was falling
apart.
There had to be something I could do, some way to do my part.
I sat and realized I had two options; act or pout.
I could sit and cry and whine that there was no way out,
Or, I could get up, wipe my face, and take some action.
But, I was only one of two; God was the rest of that fraction.
And I thought,
I will make it through with the help of God and my determination,
Even with the odds against me, I will beat discrimination (2x).
I had to show my parents the worth of their sacrifices.
So, I prayed that God would deliver us from this crisis.
I promised myself I'd graduate from a university,
And that I would show the world that good can come from diversity.
So, now I sit in class, less than six months to go.
Then, I can work more and provide my family with dough.
We've applied for residency, but that's also expensive.
And the background investigations, man those things are extensive.

But hey, we've got nothing to hide, so we should be OK.
But this process takes forever, wish it was complete today.
And it's $200 to process the first three forms.
Make sure to bend our knees and pray there's an immigration reform.
'cause if this process isn't over before there's a new president,
The new one might revoke any chance of becoming residents.
So, I've got to hurry up, so I can pay these fees
Because this lawyer doesn't get paid with only thanks and please.
Tell me getting a job isn't easy, yeah, it's rough out there
I won't accept the pessimism
I just crack my knuckles and, uh, flip my hair.
I declare my family's success, won't take no for an answer.
Gotta fight back, 'cause discrimination is like cancer.
Don't get me wrong, I love the U.S. come what may,
But I don't wanna live with the fear of losing my parents every single day.
You need money, a good lawyer, blah blah, I've heard it for so long,
Obstacles like broken records, playing the same old songs.
And I got people asking, "Why'd you choose, instead of working, to go to college?"
I'm not doing it for me, not just to gain knowledge.
I do it so at grad I can say "good job mom and dad,
You got me here because you gave everything you had.
My degree is for you, so are the blessings that come from it.
It's because of you I'm on top. It's because of you I've reached the summit."
So, now I'm looking up, and so darn optimistic.
Got a smile on my face, been so long, I surely missed it.
I embrace the discriminated, hyphenated me,
The Mexican-American my parents soon will be.
And as for our future,
We will make it through with the help of God, and with determination,
Even with the odds against us we will beat discrimination. (2x)

■

José's and Daisy's performances work to fulfill qualities of effective autoethnography and critical work. Each is self-reflexive of their sociopolitical interactivity placing their bodies on the line of border politics. Each is a provocative weave of story and theory that moves both emotionally and critically as they narrate lived experience in a sociocultural context. Each performance works through and emboldens the varying modes of using autoethnography as methodology (e.g., mode of research/inquiry, mode of re/presentation, mode of critique and resistance, mode of activism).

Each of the performances engages in a systematic unpacking of experience as a form of social criticism; each offers clear conclusions not designed as controls, but as possibilities of knowing and engaging the social world. And each is aesthetically pleasing and intellectually astute, demanding that the audience use these contributing qualities as information gathering, truth seeking, action steps, and templates for engaging their own situatedness of being (see Alexander, 2009). And maybe, more importantly to the particularity of this exploration, each critical autoethnographic exploration illuminates a complex intersectionality of being and becoming.

Both José and Daisy explicitly frame their autoethnographic performance as political, activist, and resistive. Daisy marks a struggle against discrimination and her particular involvement in political protest against Immigration and Customs Enforcement (ICE) in the Inland Empire (IE) of Southern California. José discusses his Mexican American masculine identity construction and the iterations of discrimination he experiences as a result. Each of these performances was a partial and self-referential tale that connected with other stories, ideas, discourses, and contexts of these performances, as well as being delivered in a class at a predominantly Hispanic Serving campus—with many first-generation, and a number of "undocumented" students in the class, who, at the end of these performances, began to narrate aspects of their own experiences. Each performance created a plausible and visceral lifeworld and a charged emotional atmosphere as an incitement to act within and outside the context of the work.

These performative engagements sought to articulate and identify the hidden forces and ambiguities that operate beneath the appearance of their story as well as keying in the nexus of the broader politics of immigration and border rhetorics. Each excavated the critical expressions and conditions of living within his or her interpretive culture, inspiring acts of justice; and by virtue of their first-person subjective location, they sought to name and analyze what is intuitively felt and expressed in the narrative. And both of these autoethnographic performances engaged in a critical dialogue with history, social structure, and culture, which the performances help to foreground as always and already dialectically revealed through action, feeling, thought, and language—with an embodied critical intersectionality of their own predicament. And maybe therein lies the complicated beauty of critical autoethnography as intersectional praxis. Both José and Daisy engage in an argument of intersectionality not exclusive on a bodily or cellular level, but acknowledging the social construction of identity—as historical, social, locational, and cultural—their bodies meeting at the borders and politics of time and place; bodies on the line in public debate of value and territorial imperatives that have human consequences (see Alexander, 2009).

The Classroom as a Border/less Frame: A Conclusion

My purpose in this short chapter was to explore an approach of teaching critical/autoethnography as an exercise in intersectionality and the ways in which the borders of identities bleed. In the process, I offered you two student examples undergirded by principles of theory that define my approach to a critical autoethnography and critical intersectionality with allusions to effective qualities in each. The work of my students engages a level of complex theorizing that forestalls, and at times brings into sharp contrast, the facile and reductive orientation of intersectionality limited by just race, gender, and class to address a more complex critical intersectionality that speaks to the politics of bleeding identities that include, among others, national and international politics of citizenship, issues of desire and disdain in which the body is revealed as always and already a political location; a nexus of being, as well as a literal and figurative border crossing. In fact, each performance is an act of resistance and a struggle for self-definition that bleeds the borders of the expected and the known—voices struggling to be heard between complex and overlapping borders of identity.

My own autoethnographic entry was presented as an intersectional study of my race and gender, the politics of legalized same sex marriage, and the bleeding borders of "brother status" in a fixed liquidity of time and space. But while I situate my autoethnography in an analysis of a photographic image of my biological brothers and myself—these variables of race, sexuality, and gender are always and already present within the dailiness of my life. They often become palpable in the classroom. The classroom as a confluence where bodies and lives, cultures, and curricula often encounter each other in a clash of determinations and destinations. The classroom, where historically, only particular stories have been told in a linear fashion that resists cultural variations of situated tellings; stories told of conquest that do not recognize the bodies of students that refuse to be colonized over and over again through someone else's narrative authority. The classroom, where the body of the teacher becomes reductively representative of the curriculum; ahistoricized, dera(c)ed, and neutered, talking a talk that often threatens to perpetuate self-oppression. And alike, the complex lives of students are made generic for the ease of transmitting a particular knowledge, often void of a critical application and recognition of how students resist facile explanations of compartmentalized realities, because often their lives, as does our own, intersect and straddle multiple bordered realities. In the classroom, I often flaunt my particularity as a teacher—as a black/gay/male teacher in the ivory tower. I flaunt it, not as gaudy evidence, but as a dissenting member to professed social constructs; like that picture of myself captured in a borderless frame standing in a tan suit next to three white tuxedoes—presumed difference in relation to orthodoxy; a photo that I staged to commemorate a moment so that I could consistently critique that reality from the inside out and from the outside in. In the classroom, I often engage in a critical show and tell. The materiality of my body and manner captured in the gaze of students, shows a sense of who I am—so I follow up with telling; critical tellings of lived experiences of growing up in the south; critical tellings of my life with my partner of fifteen years—tellings of our talks about our marriage as a resistance to public propositions that would deny us such a right. I metaphorically share with students who we would invite or not invite to our wedding, to be in our wedding, to be the best man, and why. I tell intimacies of the personal, not to titillate, but to tease at what should and should not be spoken of in the classroom—thereby sanctioning students to also tell; to tell of their tales, to tell of their travels, to tell of the tensions and the tensive aspects of their lived experiences that bring them to this current moment; experiences that cross borders but always carry the residual tracks of where they come from and how they live between worlds and realities. I like the idea of tracking and trafficking stories across the borders of the classroom.

The classroom is like a borderless frame; a series of contextualized engagements that offer the allusion of possibility but contain a particular territory, a particular reality. Critical autoethnography as critical praxis bleeds what Roger I. Simon (1992) refers to as the *horizon of possibility,* creating an "openness of expression of capacities encouraged in a free society and the normative, regulating forces of those social forms which define the terrain on which everyday life is lived" and storied (p. 28). It becomes what Aronowitz and Giroux (1991) might call a *border pedagogy* that helps students to understand that "[o]ne's class, race, gender, or ethnicity may influence, but does not irrevocably predetermine, how one takes up a particular ideology, reads a particular text, or responds to particular forms of oppression" (p. 119).

In the photographic image of my brothers and me, it may appear that I am held in a particular stasis of that relational dynamic, but that is just a photographic image. My life is much more expansive, and I wear multiple suits of different colors. I offer my students the possibilities of seeing themselves and showing themselves in such ways, in the classroom.

Note

1 This chapter was originally published under the same title in *Critical Autoethnography: Intersecting Cultural Identities in Everyday Life*, edited by Robin M. Boylorn and Mark P. Orbe, 98–110, © 2013, Left Coast Press, Inc. Reprinted here with permission.

References

Alexander, B. K. (2009). Autoethnography: Exploring modalities and sub-jectivities that shape social relations. In J. Paul, J. Kleinhammer-Tramill & K. Fowler (Eds.), *Qualitative research methods in special education* (pp. 277–334). Denver, CO: Love Press.

Alexander, B. K. (2011). Bordered and bleeding identities: An autocritogra-phy of shifting academic life. In S. Jackson & R. G. Johnson III (Eds.), *The black professorate: Negotiating a habitable space* (pp. 14–31). New York: Peter Lang Press.

Aronowitz, S., & Giroux, H. (1991). *Postmodern education: Politics, culture & social criticism*. Minneapolis: University of Minnesota Press.

Crenshaw, K. W. (1995). Mapping the margins: Intersectionality, identity, politics, and violence against women of color. In K. W. Crenshaw, N. Gotanda, C. Peller & K. Thomas (Eds.), *Critical race theory: The key writings that formed the movement* (pp. 357–383). New York: The New Press.

Lee, W. (2012). For the love of love: Neoliberal governmentality, neoliberal melancholy, critical intersectionality and the advent of solidarity with the other moments. *Journal of Homosexuality*. Downloaded August, 28, 2012. dx.doi.org/10.1080/009183 69.2012.699830

Madison, D. S. (2005). *Critical ethnography: Methods, ethics, and performance*. Thousand Oaks, CA: Sage.

Simon, R. I. (1992). *Teaching against the grain: Texts for a pedagogy of possibility*. New York: Bergin & Garvey.

Spry, T. (2011). *Body, paper, stage: Writing and performing autoethnography*. Walnut Creek, CA: Left Coast Press, Inc.

Chapter 7

Writing Myself into *Winesburg, Ohio*

Laura Atkins

In the beginning when the world was young there were a great many thoughts but no such thing as a truth. Man made the truths himself and each truth was a composite of a great many vague thoughts. All about in the world were the truths and they were all beautiful. ... And then the people came along. Each as he appeared snatched up one of the truths and some who were quite strong snatched up a dozen of them. It was the truths that made the people grotesques.... The moment one of the people took one of the truths to himself, called it his truth, and tried to live his life by it, he became a grotesque and the truth he embraced became a falsehood.

(Sherwood Anderson, *Winesburg, Ohio*)

Life in a Small Town

Winesburg, Ohio is a 1919 collection of short stories by Sherwood Anderson. The fictional town of Winesburg is largely based on the writer's memories of his own childhood town of Clyde, Ohio. Winesburg provides a picturesque setting for Anderson's

Qualitative Inquiry and the Politics of Research edited by Norman K. Denzin and Michael D. Giardina, 159–175.

stories—a quaint rural Ohio community reminiscent of an earlier time when people farmed and owned independent businesses. While the time period is post-Civil War, Anderson describes Winesburg as being excluded from the social and cultural influences of the industrial revolution. Each short story examines the life of a Winesburg character, and exposes his or her private troubles and vulnerabilities. Loneliness, restlessness, disillusionment, and isolation are a few of the prevailing themes of these stories that paint a picture of a town composed of disenfranchised inhabitants.

Like the characters in Winesburg, residents in present-day Clyde have a long history of family ties to the town. It is an 'everybody knows everybody' type of community. Residents will describe the many selling points to small town living—Clyde provides safety, a peaceful lifestyle, beautiful nature, and is a place where one would want to raise children. It is reminiscent of a 1950s identity. Many have fond memories of growing up in the old-fashioned small town atmosphere of Clyde:

> There was a candy store where you walk in and buy your penny candy. We collected pop bottles…turned 'em in at the carry-out for money to go to the candy store. Pretty much everybody knew everybody… Almost the same as it is today except our downtown is pretty much gone anymore, like most places. (Erika)

> Neighborhood kids would always play together. Uh, always went to Whirlpool Park—swimming. We just, seemed like we had a lot more fun than kids today have, I mean self-imposed fun, you know. We'd build wooden race cars, and race 'em down the hills, on the streets and our street was all brick. But it just, I always enjoyed it. (Carl)

Residents describe their continuing love for Clyde. As one 69-year-old woman explained:

> This is our home. I've always liked Clyde and what they stand for. They're very supportive of the schools, what the kids do. I mean, it's a nice, nice little town. I love going out to the parades. It's so much fun. They have all kinds of parades, different parades at different times of the year. (Betty)

Another source of pride is connected to the economic stability of the town, provided by Whirlpool Corporation, a plant which manufactures appliances. Whirlpool Corporation is an industrial complex that is larger than the downtown area itself. It employs about 3,000 residents from Clyde, a community of approximately 6,500, and the surrounding area, making Clyde a place where it is "easy to find a job."

> I was in the Navy four years during the Korean War and I couldn't wait to get back to Clyde. And I knew I would never move. I'd starve to death before I'd ever move outta Clyde. And it is still a great community. Low, low crime. You got a big police department. I mean we probly had all the first wheelchair ramps on all the sidewalks in town before anybody ever saw them. I mean it's just that, ya know—it's the town of Whirlpool. We got everything because of Whirlpool. (George)

The presence of Whirlpool permeates the town, reinforcing the importance of Whirlpool to Clyde's identity. The company is cited with pride on community web pages. A local community pub features a "Whirlpool pork sandwich" on its menu.

As idyllic as the descriptions of the town appear, Clyde has undergone dramatic challenges since *Winesburg, Ohio* was written, most notably related to its recent classification as a cancer cluster. Since the mid-1990s, approximately 40 children have been diagnosed with or died of brain cancer and other diseases. As is often the case in disease cluster communities, environmental contaminants have been implicated as a cause of illness within Clyde, yet health agencies have had difficulty pinpointing the exact source. Collaboration between residents and public officials has been difficult, if not contentious, with regard to efforts to determine the cause of disease. An ongoing source of tension within the community exists among the residents as well, as some place blame on the Whirlpool Corporation plant while others strongly stand beside the company's denial of culpability. From 1953 to 2008 Whirlpool owned Whirlpool Park, a recreational park built by the corporation. This family-friendly space was open to relatives and friends of Whirlpool workers, providing a source of entertainment with its pool, basketball court, and playground. It also

162 ■ *Laura Atkins*

promoted a sense of exclusivity among Whirlpool workers and their families that, in the words of one resident, "made outsiders want to be a part of it."

In 2005, the Sandusky County Department of Public Health began receiving calls from residents who were concerned about the number of children developing cancer. In 2007, the local and state health departments determined that cancers of the brain and the central nervous system were significantly higher than the number of expected cases among those aged 0-19 years. From 2008 to 2011, the Ohio EPA sampled groundwater, bodies of water, and soil, and monitored the air. They did not detect chemicals that exceeded health-based standards and found no evidence of industrial contamination. In 2008, the Whirlpool Corporation closed Whirlpool Park and sold the land. In November 2012, residents stumbled upon an online report compiled by the US EPA two months earlier citing the discovery of nine feet of toxic sludge containing PCBs in the soil at the park (EPA, 2012). Whirlpool is denying responsibility for the dumping, and conducted its own tests of the site under the supervision of the US EPA, clearing itself of any wrongdoing. My entry into the field coincided with two class action lawsuits filed against Whirlpool Corporation in March 2013, one of which is proceeding to federal court. While the company refused to allow victims to have the sites in question independently tested, Whirlpool's vice president of communications and public affairs said, "We understand where the families are coming from. We have great empathy for the families. Our issue is with attorneys who have used no science, no fact" (Henry 2013).

Science, Health, and "Will-o'-the-Wisp" Things

The detrimental effects of toxin exposure on health have been well documented. Maternal and child health are the most vulnerable to environmental toxins. It is worth noting that some leading scholars frame the issue of environmental health as a women's rights issue. Researchers have found associations between air pollutants and chemical exposure and adverse pregnancy outcomes, including preterm delivery, the leading cause of perinatal mortality (Berhman & Butler, 2006; Chen et al., 2002; Leem et al.,

2006; Maisonet et al., 2004; Maroziene & Grazuleviciene, 2002; Wilhelm & Ritz, 2003). Because the placenta is unable to block most synthetic chemicals stored in a woman's body fat, chemicals have the ability to cause subtle damage to the developing fetus, repercussions of which may manifest in the form of behavioral and cognitive problems, as well as birth defects (Hurst et al., 2002). Up to 300 synthetic chemicals have been found in body fat and in breast milk (Del Rio Gomez & Campaigns, 2007).

The most rapid periods of growth occur in utero, during infancy, and during puberty (Wargo, 1998). These periods of accelerated growth, which involve an increase in the number of cells in the body, are also periods of heightened sensitivity to toxic substances (Wargo, 1998). In addition to having higher rates of cell proliferation, which are positively correlated with an increased susceptibility to carcinogens, children have less developed detoxifying mechanisms (Wargo, 1998). A child's body composition, the proportion of body weight made up of fat tissue, and the distribution of fat may also have an important influence on childhood risks from pesticides (Wargo, 1998).

Yet another reason that children are more vulnerable to toxins than adults lies in the fact that some toxins, referred to as "initiators," are not capable of inducing tumors alone, but are believed to require later exposure to chemical "promoters," "which further alter the genetic code governing cell reproduction" (Wargo, 1998). Thus, exposure to toxins during childhood increases the probability that the initiated cells will be "promoted through additionally necessary stages of tumor development," given that a child has a longer period of time during which exposure to promoters may occur (Wargo, 1998, p. 176).

Despite an abundance of literature that supports the link between toxins and disease, much scientific inquiry is still considered "preliminary." Subject to the whims of political influence, science, health, and risk are shaped by political and economic relationships. This is generally exemplified, as in the case of Clyde, by the political resistance to investigate disease clusters and the slow response from the local, state, and federal governments.

In 2012, Robert Indian, chief of the state's comprehensive cancer-control program at the Ohio Department of Health, announced that the department would take a "very 21ˢᵗ-century" approach to cancer—one that involved avoiding time spent on cancer cluster cases whenever possible and spending more time boosting prevention and early detection of disease. "There's more payoff in that, and it does more good than continuing to pursue these will-o'-the-wisp things," he said. Cancer-cluster investigations "use a lot of resources, raise expectations, and you find nothing" (Crane, 2012).

Ohio has suffered from a number of confirmed disease clusters, two of which have directly impacted children. Located in central Ohio, the Village of Wellington is another one of five disease clusters in the state. In the mid-1990s, the Ohio EPA began receiving complaints from Wellington residents regarding dust fallout and odors from the Sterling Foundry, a facility that produced gray and ductile iron castings, primarily for heavy industry (2005). Shortly after these complaints were made, Wellington residents began to raise concerns about environmental toxins and the high rates of illness within their community. A 1998 study by the Ohio Department of Health and the Lorain County Health Department, which used data from the National Health Interview Survey, identified that residents there were 3.7 times more likely to develop Multiple Sclerosis (MS) than the rest of the country. Although the causes of MS are unknown, it is a lifelong chronic disease believed to stem from both genetic and environmental factors. Wellington residents have also expressed concerns about cancer, fibromyalgia, and lupus within their community.

In the late 1990s in Marion County, Ohio, residents began questioning the high cancer rates among graduates of the River Valley schools. The Ohio EPA discovered that the high school and middle school were built on a former army waste dump where students could have been exposed to more than 75 hazardous contaminants. After families fought to close the schools, the district relocated the schools three miles away. However, the state health department ended the investigation of 83 leukemia cases after five years without determining a cause because of a lack of direct evidence that the chemicals caused the cancer (Barry, 2013).

Indian's comment of disease clusters as "will-o-the-wisp things" conveyed a defeatist, passive attitude that was disconcerting to the families in Clyde fighting to find answers on behalf of their children. From the perspective of one mother I interviewed whose eleven-year-old daughter had passed away, it meant "we don't wanna find out."

Despite his insensitivity and poorly chosen words, there is some truth to Indian's statement. In one way, scientific methods are not very successful with regard to conveying the level of threat posed by carcinogens to communities (Edwards, 2009). It has been shown that when compounds interact with one another, toxic effects can be more harmful than those resulting from singular exposure (Wargo, 1998). However, when testing chemicals for their potential danger to human health or determining acceptable limits of exposure, the US regulatory system considers them in isolation from each other and does not account for the transformation of these compounds via interaction. The unwillingness to consider the effects of compounding chemicals further delays efforts towards the prevention of disease. Furthermore, determining the causal effect of a single toxin on health is challenging because individuals are exposed to a complex mixture of carcinogenic compounds throughout their lifetimes. It is very difficult to predict exposure to the substances now presumed to be a complex mixture of initiators and promoters (Wargo, 1998). The complex analysis of health disparities research also makes interpretation of results difficult. Conservative cut-offs for statistical significance mean that disease clusters in small communities may be overlooked, and consequently, opportunities are lost for creating meaningful policy (Diez-Roux, 1998).

Though not included in the public health assessments conducted in this area, it is of interest that many adults in the community of Clyde have also been affected by illness and disease. For example, many adult residents have presented with an inordinate number of unusual and multiple cancers, including spine cancer, eye tumors, and cancer of the spleen. Their lack of inclusion in public health assessments highlights a lack of scrutiny in the US regulatory system, and the limited resources directed to research, tracking, and prevention. Under the current model, communities across the United States carry the burden of proving that a substance is dangerous.

I entered the field in March 2013 when results from independent environmental tests indicated higher levels of Benzaldehyde in the dust of affected Clyde families' attics, an indication to scientists that other hazardous chemicals may have once been present. Over the course of five weeks, I rented a room in the home of a family in Clyde and conducted 30 interviews with residents between the ages of 19 and 76 who lived proximate to the identified boundaries for the cancer cluster. I listened to residents citing their own forms of evidence. One woman shared her eyewitness accounts of dumping at Whirlpool Park:

> Well, I'm not an analyst—I didn't analyze those chemicals, but there *were* chemicals. I was suspicious. I used to run out there and say, 'what are you doing?!' I never did photograph the trucks. I wasn't out to get anybody—I've never been that kind of a person. (Josephine)

Erika, who has worked at Whirlpool for 37 years, shared with me her suspicions about occupational hazards at the Whirlpool facility. She also cited anecdotal evidence of the corporation appropriating the community's natural resources and using them to distribute waste without consent from the community:

> I have worked at Whirlpool for 37 years, and my best friend from the time I was four, she developed breast cancer at 34, and she worked at Whirlpool. I mean, this was before anything about the cancer cluster. She said, 'I think it was some of the chemicals that I worked with, in paint and porcelain.' And of course, I had always heard rumors at work that Whirlpool dumped in the creek out there just to get rid of stuff without having to pay to have it hauled away. I heard it from guys who were told to do it. And then when I was about six, my dad and I would go mushroom huntin' just west of town right outside the city limits. There used to be an apple orchard and back in one corner there was a bunch of old barrels. They were green, with different colored stuff coming out of 'em, and my dad would say, 'don't go back there.' It was one of [Whirlpool's] dumping grounds and my dad was employed at Whirlpool for probably 40 years. So I remember from back then, him saying that stuff was there. And then there was that place on Main Street that a friend of

mine grew up in, and my dad said Whirlpool had buried barrels in their front yard.... So when all these kids started gettin' it, and they said it could be the PCBs and all that. Then I kind of started wondering if what my girlfriend—'cause my girlfriend eventually died in 2000—I thought, I wonder if that odd comment she made back then really was true.

The Truth of Community

Interviews with residents in present-day Clyde indicate a more complicated, but similarly inharmonious community to that of the fictional town of Winesburg. As if the burden of proof weren't difficult enough to contend with, families searching for answers face dissension by many residents in the community, which is exacerbated by conflicting information from government agencies. After the lawyer of the families and his team released their Benzaldehyde findings—a chemical defined as a hazardous substance by the EPA—the Ohio Department of Health released an informational sheet stating that the chemical is non-toxic, commonly found in food and household items. Graphics on the flyer included a colorful arrangement of gumballs, a ripe bundle of cherries, a bountiful harvest of fruit, a tray of baked goods, and a cup of frozen yogurt—illustrations symbolic of good times and pleasantly reminiscent of innocence and youth. While the type of graphics added to this particular fact sheet may be surprising to some, the illustrations on this example are not an out-of-the-ordinary model for fact sheets that the Ohio Department of Health has released in the past. However, one might speculate as to the timing of the release of the informational sheet, which was quickly and widely distributed. It was published in the local newspaper, and according to one woman I interviewed, it was even handed out at the building where residents pay utility bills.

Residents who advocated for Whirlpool's innocence were quick to cite the document in my interviews with them. The politics of the issue is exacerbated by the community's loyalty to Whirlpool, the company that has employed sometimes three generations of their family members. Among the "pro-Whirlpool" supporters, as residents refer to them, there is concern that Whirlpool will close, which will devastate the community. Some residents consider

Whirlpool a "good neighbor," a point reinforced by the personifi-
cation of the company. Tom, a 52-year-old banker, explained that
even if Whirlpool were cleared of responsibility, Whirlpool might
leave the town anyway because the company would feel "hurt" that
the community turned on them.

For many, to threaten Whirlpool is to threaten the community itself. When asked how such elevated rates of cancer in such
a small area could be explained, a number of possible explanations were cited, including the possibility of legacy chemicals
from prior agricultural use and industries. Some explained cancer
as "in the genes" and an "act of god." The prevalence of illness at
the Whirlpool facility was described as an expected occupational
hazard. Others similarly discounted evidence of mass occurrence
of cancer by generalizing cancer as inevitable and something that
would occur anyway. Julie, a 50-year-old bookkeeper, explained
that "other places have hurricanes, and more tornadoes than we
have, and so there are other forms of problems. God's kinda got
a plan for you and it's gonna get you no matter where you're at."

Some lamented about the stigma of being labeled a "cancer
cluster town." It was not uncommon for non-residents to question
members of the community about their decision to stay in Clyde.
To this question, many explained their long-standing ties to the
community and their love for Clyde. Barb, who suffers from
Crohn's Disease, explained:

> How do you answer that? I don't know. It's kinda like the
> Oklahoma people. They're coming out of their storm shelters.
> And well, you know, we're Oklahomans what can you do? We're
> gonna stay here.

Parents of children who are ill or have died cited the same reasons
for staying in Clyde. Brian, whose two children are in remission
from leukemia, adds to this discussion two additional concerns—
the financial burden of managing illness, an obvious concern,
and an effort to maintain a sense of normalcy for his children.
In his words:

> Everything else has been taken away from them so we wanted
> to do everything we could to keep our home because they were
> away in the hospital and when they came home we wanted them

to come home to *home*. Because everything else was different—
they pretty much grew apart from their friends because you don't
have all that contact with them every day and even when you do
get back to school, people treat them differently. They're different, you know, they don't have hair, they're sick a lot and miss a
lot of school, so the home thing was important to us. I mean you
have jobs, you have social ties, and you want to do everything to
protect yours, kid but at that point we don't really know what we
were protecting our kids from. So do you move them out of the
school system again further away from their friends and their
support system?

Many acknowledged that they cannot take for granted that they
can wake up and have a "normal" life anymore, perhaps one of the
selling points of small town living. Disease and contamination, or
even just the perception of contamination, have devastated a lot of
people in the community. Their quality of life has been challenged
as they confront concerns about what might be in their water, air,
and the soil around their homes. Their ability to enjoy their homes
has been compromised, and they are concerned about the health
of their children and families. Environmental contaminants
affect lifestyle choices—people's way of living, including their
pattern of activities and the relationships and places needed to
sustain these activities. Karen, whose family lives near Whirlpool
Park, laments the fact that their family memories are now tainted
with suspicions of toxin exposure. Karen and her family have been
affected by developmental delays and cognitive disorders, diver-
ticulitis, colon cancer, breast cancer, infertility, and ovarian cysts.
Even their family dogs have had a history of seizures. In reflecting
upon the park, Karen recalls:

> It was just, it was great. I mean people used to envy us because
> we lived so close to Whirlpool Park—because it was so conve-
> nient. It would be so crowded in the summertime so we'd wait
> until just about dinnertime because we always ate early. My
> [mother-in-law] always had supper on the table when her hus-
> band came in 'cause he farmed so they had a specific amount of
> time for him to eat and get back out in the field. So then I just
> kinda carried that on, and we'd already have our supper ate and

we'd go over there by the time everybody was leaving to go home and eat and then it wouldn't be crowded at all [laughs]. It's too bad that your memories are being, you know, tarnished. Because now it's like when I think about when I had my son's birthday party over there, and all my nieces and nephews were over there in the creek gathering up the frogs...I mean you just think, I don't know—were we safe or weren't we?

Beyond lifestyle, Michael Edelstein (2004) argues that contamination affects normal assumptions about life, what he terms "lifescape." That is, toxic exposure directly assails fundamental social beliefs. These include that humans hold dominion over nature, people control their own destiny, technology and science are positive and progressive forces, experts know best, and government exists to help (Edelstein, 2004). Such beliefs may also ring true for many residents of Clyde, evidenced by the many who deny, rationalize, or ignore issues of contamination to maintain their existing beliefs. However, it is also subtly detectable among those who express a sense of surprise and outrage that their rights have been trampled on. Marilyn, a 64-year-old breast cancer survivor, is confounded by the slow and weak response to the problem:

> They don't wanna be accountable for hurting anyone or be responsible for fixing the problem or to accept responsibility for creating the problem, and that's what makes it so difficult for *we the people* that don't have the education to know who to contact, how to know what questions to ask, how to understand the question that was asked and understand what it meant. Somewhere along the line somebody has got to be accountable for that. A *good neighbor*'s gotta stop and say, 'Hey we did that. You're darn right, we're gonna clean it up.' That's a good neighbor. And I'm a big one in *made in America*. I'm very patriotic. I'm very much a USA girl... [I] think it's just *we the people* are lost here somewhere, we're just lost. I don't know how you get it back, how do you get it back? You have children die to get it back?

From these narratives, there is a sense that the whole meaning of "small town Clyde" and all of its real and imagined charms are threatened. From some residents, it seems as if there is a romanticized and nostalgic perception of a community identity similar to those of days gone by. Yet, like the other social beliefs residents hold onto, many remain loyal to the small town identity in spite of the fact that, under current circumstances, it is being challenged.

Meanwhile, Clyde is adapting to cancer as a way of life. Cancer fundraisers have become commonplace community events that many people attend. The town has become very efficient at hosting these and raising significant amounts of money for affected families. From chicken or spaghetti dinners to auctions, the fundraisers give residents a way to be proactively involved and help buffer the financial hardships that victims face. Erika explains:

> I always buy all the t-shirts. I try to get involved and help 'cause I know the bills are horrible and that they just can't...like Emily... her mom's been up at the hospital with her I think since the day she went in. She's been there ninety-some days and she works at Whirlpool. I don't know if they gave her a leave of absence or what, but you know you don't wanna leave your fourteen-year-old or any child that is going through this by themselves because they need help in all kinds of ways.

Fundraisers have become so commonplace that they have redefined what it means to be a part of the community. Residents are proud of the outpouring of compassion and participation. Among the residents, this is perceived as a normal response to the systemic emotional impact of cancer diagnosis within a close-knit community. Some residents describe the fundraisers, which occur nearly every weekend, as social events unique to the community. As Carl explains, "It's like if ya haven't been to a fundraiser or don't have a wristband, then you're not in *our* community." Sometimes the tickets sell out so quickly that the residents have to wait for the next event to attend.

In addition to the fundraisers, other evidence of support is present within the community. Cancer stickers adorn cars. Tip jars are placed on the counters of restaurants and other businesses to collect money in support of cancer research. Every school year, the elementary students have "cancer week," and each day of the week they wear a different colored ribbon representing a different type of cancer. There are cancer centers and radiation treatment facilities throughout the town, including a Cleveland Clinic Cancer Center adjacent to Whirlpool. Parents, physicians, and school nurses are more vigilant to signs of illness.

All of these responses have been accepted as the new norm in Clyde. To an outside observer, it is not natural that the community would have to adapt in the ways that it has. There is a sense of defeat that is attached to their acceptance, a probable consequence of the lack of response and resolution to contamination. These activities empower residents because the activities make them feel like they are doing something helpful. Also attached to this acceptance is a lingering "we the people" sentiment—namely, an unwillingness to let go of the belief that someone is looking out for them, and that correct behavior will win the day. In a more subtle way, these activities provide a venue through which small town values are preserved, including accepting the community problems as one's own. Yet it falls short in that it diverts attention from other forms of activism and dilutes efforts towards finding the proper resolution that would lead to cleaning up the problem and making their town safe again.

An Inconclusive Story

The fictional town of Winesburg was full of characters that operated independently, each facing his or her private turmoil that could not be overcome. The conflict that residents in present-day Clyde face is relatable to the isolation and hopelessness of those stories. Regardless of where residents stand as to the causes of illness within the community, those impacted experience a great deal of turmoil over the issue. No one has really stepped in to find answers or correct the problem. Nor has anyone been held accountable, and residents have been left with few resources to solve the problem on their own. Consequently, their versions of truth, community, and hope have been degraded. People who preferred a small town, and perhaps idyllic life, are facing a catastrophe wherein children are dying, neighbors mistrust each other, there is a lack of faith in the government, residents are financially burdened, and the community is fearful of the future. As diverse as my interviews were, there was a common thread among them—people's definition of their place in their world is changing.

Like most of the characters in Winesburg who are portrayed in moments of crisis, my interviews have exposed vulnerable moments with Clyde residents. One interaction that resonated with me occurred during an interview with a woman who had survived four bouts with cancer when she lived near Whirlpool Park. As traumatic as those events could be, her biggest burden, however, seemed to be the suicide of her veteran son. During my visit to her home, she led me into a room to show me her baby—a life-like doll. "Look at her little feet," she said. "Smell her. I say goodnight to her, you know. I've always loved babies. Look at her little hands." She insisted that I hold the baby. I held it awkwardly for a minute, and then I rocked the baby. I could feel her weight in the muscles of my arms. I held her confidently as we stood together in a shared experience of different kinds of loneliness. Moments like these have made me realize that we all—sociologists and anthropologists alike—have a place in *Winesburg, Ohio*.

On the cover of *Winesburg, Ohio* is a painting by Andrew Wyeth called "Christina's World." It portrays a woman lying on the ground in a treeless field, looking up at a gray house on the horizon. The woman in the painting, Christina Olson, suffered from polio—a muscular deterioration that paralyzed her lower body. Wyeth was inspired to create the painting when, watching from a window in his house, he saw her crawling across a field. The selection of this painting for the cover of *Winesburg, Ohio* couldn't have been more appropriate. It not only captures the metaphorical disability of the characters, it almost stands as a foretelling of events that were yet to come in the real town of Clyde. The feeling of isolation in the painting is woven into both stories. In one way, I am like Wyeth in the window—quietly captivated by how others manage their vulnerabilities. In yet another way, I can empathize with Christina—struggling outside of the text, in the textured field of qualitative inquiry, edging closer to an understanding.

References

Anderson, S. (1919). *Winesburg, Ohio.* New York: B. W. Huebsch.

Agency for Toxic Substances and Disease Registry. (2005). "Health consultation: Village of wellington." Retrieved October 15, 2012, from www.atsdr.cdc.gov/hac/pha/VillageofWellington031705OH/VillageofWellington031705-OH.pdf

Barry, A. (2013, May 14). Return to River Valley: Some families still believe school grounds led to cancer. 10TV.com (Columbus). Retrieved April 12, 2014, from www.10tv.com/content/stories/2013/05/13/marion-return-to-river-valley-cancer-concerns.html

Berhman, R. E., & Butler, A. S. (2006). *Preterm birth: Causes, consequences, and prevention. Report from the Institute of Medicine's Committee on Understanding Premature Birth and Assuring Healthy Outcome.* Washington, D.C.: National Academies Press.

Chen, L.,Yang, W., Jennison, B. L., Goodrich, A., & Stanly, T. (2002). Air pollution and birth weight in Northern Nevada, 1991–1999. *Inhalation Toxicology, 14*(2), 141–157.

Crane, M. (2012, June 11). State wary of cancer clusters but will continue investigations. The *Columbus Dispatch.* Retrieved February 10, 2015, from www.dispatch.com/content/stories/local/2012/06/11/state-no-longer-examines-cancer-clusters.html

Del Rio Gomez, I., & Campaigns, L. E. (2007). *Gender and environmental chemicals.* London: Women's Environmental Network.

Diez-Roux, A. V. (1998). Bringing context back into epidemiology: Variables and fallacies in multilevel analysis. *American Journal of Public Health, 88*(2), 216–222.

Edelstein, M. (2004). *Contaminated communities,* 2/e. Boulder, CO: Westview.

Edwards, N. (2008). An ounce of precaution. *Contexts, 7*(20), 26–30.

Henry, T. (2013, November 1). Whirlpool contractor exonerates Clyde site. The *Toledo Blade.* Retrieved February 10, 2015, from www.toledoblade.com/local/2013/11/01/Whirlpool-contractor-exonerates-Clyde-site.html

Hurst, C. H., Abbott, B., Schmid, J. E., & Birnbaum, L. S. (2002). 2,3,7,8-Tetrachlorodibenzo-p-dioxin (TCDD) disrupt early morphogenetic events that form the lower reproductive tract in female rat fetuses. *Toxicological Sciences, 65*(1), 87–98.

Leem, J., Kaplan, B. M., Shim, Y. K., Pohl, H. R., Gotway, C. A., Bullard, S. M., Rogers, J. F., Smith, M. M., & Tylenda, C. A. (2006). Exposure to air pollutants during pregnancy and preterm delivery. *Environmental Health Perspectives, 114*(6), 905–910.

Maisonet, M., Correa, A., Misra, D., & Jaakkola, J. J. (2004). A review of the literature on the effects of ambient air pollution on fetal growth. *Environmental Research, 95*(1), 6–12.

Maroziene, L., & Grazuleviciene, R. (2002). Maternal exposure to low-level air pollution and pregnancy outcomes: A population-based study. *Environmental Health, 1*(1), 1–13.

Ohio EPA, Division of Drinking and Ground Waters. (2009). *Drinking water quality sampling to support the Ohio Department of Health childhood cancer investigation, City of Clyde and surrounding townships.* Retrieved November 26, 2014, from epa.ohio.gov/portals/47/citizen/clyde/Final_Clyde_WQ_Report_041609.pdf

US EPA. *Site Assessment Report for the Whirlpool Park Site Green Springs, Sandusky County, Ohio.* Weston Solutions, Inc. 2012. Retrieved May 14, 2014. (www.epa.gov/.../cleanup/easternsandusky/pdfs/whirlpool_sa_report.pdf)

Wargo, J. (1998). *Our children's toxic legacy: How science and law fail to protect us from pesticides.* New York: Yale University Press.

Wilhelm M., & Ritz, B. (2003). Residential proximity to traffic and adverse birth outcomes in Los Angeles County, California, 1994–1996. *Environmental Health Perspectives, 111*(2), 207–216.

Wyeth, A. (1948). *Christina's World* (Painting). Currently on display at the Museum of Modern Art. New York.

Chapter 8

The Three Rs: Remembering, Revisiting, and Reworking

How We Think, but Not in School

Patrick J. Lewis

The human creature is storied. The human mind, as Jonathan Gottschall (2012) said, is "shaped *for* story, so that it could be shaped *by* story" (p. 56). It is an entwinement that makes it almost impossible to distinguish between what is a narrative mode of thought and what is a narrative text or discourse. As Jerome Bruner (1996) noted so long ago, "just as thought becomes inextricable from the language that expresses it and eventually shapes it… our experience of human affairs come to take the form of the narrative we use in telling about them" (p. 132). There is a wide and growing body of research literature across multiple disciplines that increasingly supports the idea of what Mark Turner (1997) once called the "literary mind." We live, breathe, drink, and even dream story; our penchant for working our narrative imaginations has no known boundaries. No matter how far removed something may be from our experience we will try to make sense of it through narrative imagining; we will project some kind of narrative upon it in our never ending endeavour to make sense of the world. It is how we are/think the world. Narrative imagining has both ontological and epistemological implications in our becoming and being human.

Qualitative Inquiry and the Politics of Research edited by Norman K. Denzin and Michael D. Giardina, 177–188. © 2015 Left Coast Press, Inc. All rights reserved.

Yet, if story is so central to human understanding, why then in primary schooling (Pre-k to 3) is there such a dearth of stories; they have been replaced by something called early literacy learning that manifests through levelled reading books void of simple plot or denouement. Dwayne Huebner (1999/1987) once said that teaching is a vocation, a calling; one is called by children and youth and in that process a teacher answers the call in order to be present and listen a child's story into being, to fit one chapter into her life. But, how can a teacher realize that chapter in a child's life when education policy is driven by utilitarian notions of learning to read and write with an efficiency model focused on phonics and phonemic awareness to instil decoding skills into children and then measuring them on test after test in order to increase scores? Much of the efficient literacy drive has been informed through the research of psychology, psycholinguistics, biomedical approach and the behavioral sciences. Unfortunately, "the bewitching language of psychology and the behavioral sciences has skewed our view of education" (Huebner, 1999/1993, p. 404). From the beginnings of child development and learning studies to the present the theory of developmental norms has shifted from "description to prescription: from a mythic norm (mythic because no one actually 'fits' it) to statements of how people should be" (Dahlberg & Moss, 2005, p. 7), and if a child's learning and developmental growth fall outside that prescribed trajectory, he or she may be deemed broken. What kind of story is that?

In 2007 a book I wrote was published with part of the title of this piece, *How we Think, but not in School: a storied approach to teaching*. I thought I was being clever with the 'How we think' part, because it is the title of one of John Dewey's many published works and likely one of his most important. Needless to say, I think I am the only person who knows that bit of cleverness. In that work I presented an argument for the importance of story and play in the lives of young children as they enter pre-school and primary school and the need to think about something I termed "transitional reciprocity between oracy and literacy—the movement back and forth between oral and print narrative understanding, as children learn to read and write" (Lewis, 2007, p. 46). In remembering, revisiting, and reworking this idea I have come to realize that I haven't changed my ideas much since then. In fact, probably the opposite has happened, with all the research that has been carried out with how central narrative imagining is to human cognition I believe in my thesis even more. However, what I am coming to see more clearly is the notion of play and story or play and narrative as not so much symbiotic as I suggested then, but it transcends that to a far deeper, more dynamic relationship; the one cannot exist without the other. That is, without Play there is no story and without Story there is no play, and what is born from the two is imagination; that is to say, "before play there is no imagination" (Vygotsky, as cited in El'konin, 2005, p. 14). The integration of play and story I am proposing draws in part upon Vygotsky's notion of the social origins and nature of human cognitive development and learning. As Nicolopoulou (2007) has urged, "We ought to approach children's play and narrative as closely intertwined, and often overlapping, forms of socially situated symbolic action—and that one source of valuable theoretical resources for grasping the interplay between the two is Vygotsky's sociocultural analysis of children's play" (p. 117). The primary form of play of which I am speaking is role play, that is, dramatic, sociodramatic, make-believe or pretend play; however, some rule play, constructional play, or functional play may enter or overlap.

What needs to be emphasized is that "play is the signature of childhood. It's a living, visible manifestation of imagination and learning in action" (Gopnik, 2009, p. 14). Vygotsky theorized that imagination is manifested externally through play and that imagination begins to form and develop when a child is very young, and as imagination continues to grow and develop through play it migrates inward and becomes play across the interior landscape of the psyche. He posited that for the school age child, play becomes interiorized through inner speech—and at times private speech (internal speech spoken aloud), logical memory, and abstract thought—"imagination begins to develop through play" (Vygotsky, as cited in El'konin, 2005, p. 14). Building upon Vygotsky's idea perhaps we can see narrative, play, and imagination as forming a triad in the cognitive-social-emotional development of the child and integral to early childhood learning and teaching (Pre-k to 3).

However, in our current schooling practice we tend to marginalize play and the accompanying notion of narrative and imagination to a space and time when the important work is completed, if we allow it at all. Part of what has evolved in K–12 education is the desire to define and sequence teaching and learning so that they are controlled and measured in a linear and known manner, suggesting that all is certain, including the future, but nothing could be further from the truth. In the current "race to the top," our efforts to leave no child behind through various forms of standardized assessment and prescriptive forms of literacy instruction toward "basic literacy" skills by grade 3 we are actually laying the groundwork for disengagement from school by children and most certainly are not nurturing children's imaginations. What contributes to that is our failure to "take advantage of a time in children's lives when narrative imagination and metaphoric understandings are open and willing to be stimulated" (Lewis, 2007, p. 46). As Kieran Egan has noted, a "clear understanding of children's orality is essential if we are to make what we want to teach engaging and meaningful; orality entails valuable forms of thought that need to be developed as the foundation for a sophisticated literacy" (Egan, 1999a, p. 33). Early school experience can enlarge children's learning through educational activities grounded in the principal forms of human thinking—play and story.

In oral cultures storytelling has been the central form of teaching for millennia, with children and adults enveloped in the stories of the culture through the rhythm and the rhyme of the language. Language is central in the tone, meter, images, and metaphors embodied in and through the stories of the group, the identity of the people. However, more importantly, a society's values, beliefs, and aesthetics are woven through their stories. This is also true of so-called literate societies; that is, the values and beliefs of the group pervade novels, short stories, films, television—the media in all its myriad forms, including digital citizenry. However, in oral storytelling there is

> a somatic remembering that captures the listeners' imagination so that teller and listeners transcend place to storyscape. Children, and adults, too, for that matter, when listening to

stories, are transported to the world of the story and experience the possibilities of other realities, similar [to] or very different from their own. Story allows all children, readers and nonreaders alike, to enter the story and participate in the imaginative re-creation of events containing the many and varied truths of human experience and behaviour." (Lewis, 2007, p. 76)

Listening to a story told is often an intimate experience. The listener and storyteller enter into a relationship, seeing each other live, adjusting, adapting, and moving in rhythm with the words, vocal tones, gestures, facial expressions, and movement. Consequently, story listeners, irrespective of their literacy skills or language development can enter into the oral story on their own terms. Storytelling fosters expressive language skills in both oracy and literacy, encouraging children to take up and play with new vocabulary and language in a complex, but easily understood form that we all have—story, play, and narrative imagining. Indigenous peoples know well the importance and power of story:

> In addition to developing language skills, stories teach moral lessons, convey values, and promote emotional wellness. Orality, in both skill development and meaning making on the part of the teller and the listener, is an important aspect of traditional storytelling (Weber-Pillwax, 2001).… Traditionally, meaning making was primarily the responsibility of the listener; the teller paid attention to the context and needs of the child to know which story to tell and when and how to tell it. (Goulet & Goulet, 2015, p. 18)

That storytelling and play with story does all that is extraordinary, but story does more than that. When stories are shared in relational context with children it conjures an ancient call to both the child/listener and the adult/storyteller—to respond, to act. "The act happens somewhere on the horizon of the imaginative landscape. That act, is an act of creation: the creation of possibilities and imaginative understandings in the minds of the children [and the storyteller] as the story comes alive in their present being" (Lewis, 2007, p. 76). This act of the storyteller and the listener is the "process of enthralling the audience, of impressing on them the reality of the story, [it] is a central feature of education in oral cultures…. Thus the techniques of fixing the crucial patterns of belief in the memory—rhyme, rhythm, formula, story, and so on—are vitally important" (Egan, 1999b, p. 11). Walter Benjamin (1968) said, "The first true storyteller is, and will continue to be, the teller of fairy tales" because, "whenever good counsel was at a premium, the fairy tale had it, and where the need was greatest, its aid was nearest" (p. 102). Of course today fairy tales, folk tales, parables, myths and legends are not usually given much currency. However, they persist and make themselves felt in a myriad of ways through popular culture. As Robert Scholes and Robert Kellogg (1966) noted almost half a century ago,

> once a culture loses its innocence with respect to myth, it can never recapture it. But myth, in yielding up its special characteristics, dies only to be reborn. Because mythic narrative is the expression in story form of deep-seated human concerns, fears and aspirations, the plots of mythic tales are a storehouse of narrative correlatives—keys to human psyche in story form—guaranteed to reach an audience and move them deeply. Though rationalistic attacks on myth as falsehood tend to invalidate it historically, they are powerless against its psychological potency. (Scholes & Kellogg, 1966, p. 220)

Yet, these stories should be highly valued for they give children and adults so much. Children in the primary school years (Pre-k to 3) should be immersed in folk tales, myths, and fairy tales because to do so is to engage deeply in vitally important cognitive and emotional work. When listening to a story the child "takes in the story; comprehends its sense, which is conveyed by the relations and the actions of the characters…. It is a complex internal activity" (El'koninova, 2001a, p. 40). At story time the child is not simply being entertained listening to a tale. She is engaged with an embodied experience, "a child listening to a story follows the actions of the main character with his [*sic*] inner eye; he literally feels his way through them with his whole body," emotionally experiencing and sensing "the actions of the main character as the events in the story unfold" (p. 40). This is part of the important work children do with/in story and play; it is how they "empathize and emotionally experience the events of the story as they unfold" (p. 40). Through the child's empathic emotional response to the story, the story becomes part of the child through her narrative imagining and play. "The assimilation of meaning and purpose is related to the repetitiveness of children's play" (p. 31). The child plays with stories; responding, re-acting, revising, reworking stories, through artful responses and in her desire to hear a favorite story over and over again.

The myth, the folk tale, and the fairy tale are often perceived as suitable for children because they are considered the most easily accessible narratives, seen as simple straightforward texts. Nonetheless, such tales are in fact very complicated semantically—containing "a complete system modelling the world" (El'koninova, 2001b, p. 67), but not in the way that is often construed. These tales "contain not the least clue on how to cope with undesirable behaviour, i.e., how to restrain one's selfish tendencies" (El'koninova, 2001a, p. 33). The folk tale is not a repository of examples or models of how to act ethically or lawfully. They are not exemplars of good character or moral behavior. As El'koninova found, "What the fairy tale prescribes in full aesthetic form are *models of motives* [italics added] of moral behaviour rather than models of specific ways to realize those motives, i.e., how to apply or measure up to them" (p. 34). The folk tale does not show "how the hero solves a problem, but the fact that he makes a successful decision to solve the problem, that he *decides* [italics added] to do something" (El'koninova, 2001b, p. 71). These stories are allegorical, suggesting that "if you just decide to act correctly (morally, nobly, with love), no matter what you undertake you will succeed" (p. 71).

Consequently, the play with story which children do is vitally important to their cognitive, emotional, and empathic development; the play is a process of blending which integrates the ontological and epistemological natures of story. When children engage in pretend play, re-enacting folk tales, they know they are pretending, which is demonstrative of their well developed and developing cognitive powers (Boyd, 2009, p. 181; Gopnik, 2009, pp. 29–30). Psychology once deemed children's pretend play as evidence of their inability to distinguish between fact and fiction, reality and fantasy; however, more recent research has determined this to simply be inaccurate (p. 30). As Alison Gopnik (2009) delineates in the *Philosophical Baby*, children as young as two or three years of age are capable of creating what philosophers and psychologists call counterfactuals—imagining other possible realities. Herein lies the importance of storytelling in helping children's cognitive, social, emotional and spiritual development. Story is both phenomenon and process, "counterfactuals let us change the future. Because we can consider alternative ways the world might be, we can actually act on the world and intervene to turn it into one or the other of these possibilities" (p. 23). Children play cognitively and materially with folktales; they have the story as told with the allegorical suggestion of how the principal character decides to act, and they can play with the story to explore and experience counterfactuals.

Story and play transcend place. The storyteller and the listener enter the storyscape and the player(s) enter the playscape, all the while cognizant that it is 'pretend.' But more importantly, "play is about deconstruction of context, the escape from contexts; in fact, one of play's major purposes is to make context irrelevant" (King, 1992, p. 58). Play and story are simultaneously of the material world and our inner world, the play and the story happen in the immediate place yet the play and the story transform the place into a new space in both our exterior and interior realities. Storytelling is a human universal, particularly fictional tales. "It develops spontaneously and without training in childhood in the form of pretend play" (Boyd, 2009, p. 189). There is a reciprocal cognitive entanglement with play and story from birth to death.

At this point, dear reader, if we were gathered together somewhere, perhaps with a few other people, I would demonstrate what I am trying to articulate here in this text. That is, I would tell you a story, an oral story so that we might travel into the spaces and places I have been mentioning so that you might actually experience, feel, imagine what I have been saying about story and our play with it. I could write the story here, but again that's not the same as being with a storyteller. The best I can do is provide an audio or video recording that you could listen to, but again we aren't together in the moment and in the play of story and imagination. Nevertheless, here are three links to audio–video recordings of me sharing stories with six- and seven-year-old children in a primary classroom, which hopefully will provide some insight into what I have been regaling you with in this piece.

www.youtube.com/watch?v=8wvbHRQaALY
www.youtube.com/watch?v=chk0dja6tfM
www.youtube.com/watch?v=1Sz2H6i51j0

If storytelling and play are vitally important to children's whole development, why do we not see them taken up in schools in such a way that play and story are the heart of pedagogical praxis? This is not news; Jerome Bruner (1996) showed how unaware and unknowledgeable we are about the importance of nurturing narrative understanding with children. There are two universal ideas that we must help children realize, "the first is that a child should 'know,' have a 'feel' for the myths, histories, folktales, conventional stories of his or her culture" because these are the stories that "frame and nourish an identity" (p. 41). The second is "imagination through fiction" because "finding a place in the world, for all that it implicates the immediacy of home, mate, job and friends, is ultimately an act of imagination" (p. 41). But our educational practice in the early years (Pre-k to 3) appears to have taken up the project of eroding space and time for play, story, and imagination by appealing to an adult narrative of concern, if not fear, about the literacy development of children, conventional print literacy in particular. Furthermore, there is no place for the transitional reciprocity of oracy and literacy that I advocate, "because all the energy of teaching is directed toward a narrow definition of literacy, conventional print literacy in particular and the opportunity for play; play with language and literacy is missed" (Lewis, 2007, p. 60). We neither use nor remember well enough the gift of storytelling in our pedagogical practice with children. We no longer enthral children with simple narratives full of complex knowledge about being and becoming human. Instead, we overwhelm children with literacy check lists of skills, strategies, and information of how to be a good effective reader rather than leading them into the heart of a story full of action, challenges, setbacks, decision making, problem solving, and fulfilment. We oppress with prescriptive teaching models and "tests all driving toward instilling an instrumentalist model of efficient literacy. All of this drive is based and built upon 'adult literate concepts in our pedagogy' (Herriman, 2005, p. 81) which [do not tolerate or] are insensitive to the oracy" (Lewis, 2007, p. 77) and narrative understanding of young children embodied in their play and story making.

Certainly we should be demanding more from our schools than producing people who are efficient in reading and mathematics based on an increasingly narrow notion of an efficient literacy. I am not suggesting reading and math are not important, they are indeed important, but how literacy is *defined and distributed* in current practice, policy and curriculum warrants a second look. Shouldn't we be ensuring that the early educational experiences (Pre-k to 3) of all children are built around the notion of the triad of play, story, and imagination? Dare I suggest a fourth R, "Re-imagine" instead of the endless R of "Reform"? Perhaps, we need to Re-imagine what early learning and teaching could be for children, families, teachers, and society. But of course, one is quick to ask: How might we begin such a vitally important project and what would we teach and who would decide? We might begin by transcending what Kieran Egan (1999) called the "curriculum wars" and begin by asking once again: What are the *aims* of education, not the goals, objectives, outcomes, indicators benchmarks or targets, but the aims? How might we imagine early learning and teaching with three- to eight-year-old children?

> One way this may happen is by remaking education as a reciprocal journey with teacher and child as partners, collaborators removed from the present hierarchy of school and learning; similar to Paulo Freire's (1970, 1994) desire to cultivate a deep reciprocity between teacher and child/youth. It would see a flattening of the hierarchal structure of school and learning so that teachers, children, youth and parents *care for* and have *hope with* each other. (Lewis, 2009, p. 14)

Perhaps we can begin by utilizing what I delineated about narrative understanding and imagining at the beginning of this chapter and ask: What story can we imagine for children and their families as they begin the journey alongside adults in the creation and telling of the story of their own learning journey? To embark on such a journey requires that teachers and children bring their stories into being so that the pedagogical odyssey becomes a collaborative exploration into story "where the newness and wonder that children bring to their engagement with the quotidian reminds us, parents and teachers, of the incongruences, the entanglements and the rhizomatic renderings of being" (Lewis, 2009, p. 14). In such a story the curriculum transcends current practice and is taken up by teachers and children and embodied as "their journey through life" (Huebner, 1999/1995, p. 443) experienced together through a reciprocal partnership; confronting the challenges, desires, and joys of being. To imagine this is to imagine that education can be other than, more than how it is currently lived, it can be a different story. But to live that story will require a fusion of intelligence and passion, care and empathy, and a trust amongst us all as we travel into an uncertain future. That would be a good story.

References

Benjamin, W. (1968). The storyteller: Reflections on the work of Nicolai Leskov. In W. Benjamin, *Illuminations* (pp. 83–110). Trans. H. Zorn. New York: Schocken Books.

Boyd, B. (2009). *On the origin of stories: Evolution, cognition, and fiction.* Cambridge, MA: Harvard University Press

Bruner, J. (1996). *The culture of education.* Cambridge, MA: Harvard University Press.

Dahlberg, G., & Moss, P. (2005). *Ethics and politics in early childhood education.* London: RoutledgeFalmer.

Egan, K. (1999a). Literacy and the oral foundations of education. In *Children's minds talking rabbits & clockwork oranges: Essays on education* (pp. 3–33). London, ONT: Althouse Press.

Egan, K. (1999b). Clashing armies in the curriculum wars. In *Children's minds talking rabbits & clockwork oranges: Essays on education* (pp. 93–110). London, ONT: Althouse Press.

El'konin, D. B. (2005). The psychology of play. *Journal of Russian and East European Psychology, 43*(1), 11–97.

El'koninova, L. I. (2001a). The object orientation of children's play in the context of understanding imaginary space-time in play and in stories. *Journal of Russian and East European Psychology, 39*(2), 30–51.

El'koninova, L. I. (2001b). Fairy-tale semantics in the play of preschoolers. *Journal of Russian and East European Psychology, 39*(4), 67–87.

Gopnik, A. (2009). *The philosophical baby: What children's minds tell us about truth, love and the meaning of life.* New York: Farrar, Straus and Giroux.

Gottschall, J. (2012). *The storytelling animal: How stories make us human.* New York: Mariner Books.

Goulet, L. M., & Goulet, K. N. (2015). *Teaching each other: Nehinuw concepts & Indigenous pedagogies.* Vancouver, BC: UBC Press.

Huebner, D. (1999/1987). Teaching as vocation. In V. Hillis (Ed.), *The lure of the transcendent, collected essays by Dwayne Huebner* (pp. 379–387). Mahwah, NJ: Lawrence Erlbaum Associates.

Huebner, D. (1999/1993). Education and spirituality. In V. Hillis (Ed.), *The lure of the transcendent, collected essays by Dwayne E. Huebner* (pp. 401–416). Mahwah, NJ: Lawrence Erlbaum Associates.

Huebner, D. (1999/1995). Challenges bequeathed. In V. Hillis (Ed.), *The lure of the transcendent, collected essays by Dwayne E. Huebner* (pp. 432–449). Mahwah, NJ: Lawrence Erlbaum Associates.

King, N. (1992). The impact of content on the play of young children. In S. Kessler & B. Swadener (Eds.), *Reconceptualizing the early childhood curriculum: Beginning the dialogue* (pp. 43–61). New York: Teachers College Press.

Lewis, P. (2007). *How we think, but not in school: A storied approach to teaching.* Rotterdam, NL: Sense.

Lewis, P. (2009). Who in this culture speaks for children and youth? In P. Lewis & J. Tupper (Eds.), *Challenges bequeathed: Taking up the challenges of Dwayne Huebner* (pp. 13–24). Rotterdam, NL: Sense.

Nicolopoulous, A. (2005). The interplay of play and narrative in children's development: Theoretical reflections and concrete examples. In A. Göncü & S. Gaskins (Eds.), *Play and development: Evolutionary, sociocultural, and functional perspectives.* New York: Lawrence Erlbaum.

Scholes, R., & Kellogg, R. (1966). *The nature of narrative.* London: Oxford University Press.

Turner, M. (1997). *The literary mind.* New York: Oxford University Press.

Vygotsky, L. (1933/2002). Play and its role in the mental development of the child. C. Mulholland (Trans.). In *Psychology and Marxism internet archive (marxists.org) 2002.* Retrieved May 24, 2006, from www.marxists.org/archive/vygotsky/works/1933/play.htm

Weber-Pillwax, C. (2001). What is Indigenous research? *Canadian Journal of Native Education, 25*(2), 166–174.

Chapter 9

Teaching Reflexivity in Qualitative Research

Fostering a Research Life Style

Judith Preissle and Kathleen deMarrais

Reflexivity is central to qualitative research practice, but can be challenging for students to learn and practice. Studying and documenting the researcher within the research, studying ourselves as we study our topics, participants, and settings, requires balance, discretion, and judgment. Documenting our reflexivity produces research autobiographies and subjectivity statements (DeMarrais, 1998; Preissle, 2008), accounts of our inquiries from our own viewpoints. What helps and hinders twenty-first century students in efforts to be reflexive? How do we go about this study and practice?

Requiring students to document their decisions, plans, worries, and uncertainties as they work through assignments from the beginning of their research courses and programs develops habits of reflexivity, provides practice in reflexivity, and supports learning to write reflexively. We advocate as part of our qualitative pedagogy approaching research not just as an exercise or activity or job, but also as an inquiring, mindful life style. In this presentation we address these topics.

Qualitative Inquiry and the Politics of Research edited by Norman K. Denzin and Michael D. Giardina, 189–196. © 2015 Left Coast Press, Inc. All rights reserved.

What Is Reflexivity?

Reflexivity is the practice of studying and documenting the researcher within the research: studying ourselves as we study our topics, participants, and settings. Documenting our reflexivity produces research autobiographies, accounts of our inquiries from our own viewpoints. What hinders us in our efforts to be reflexive? How do we go about this study and practice?

Qualitative traditions vary considerably, depending on the disciplines and fields that developed them. However, most traditions depend on the researcher as the central data collection method—the researcher as the instrument (Wolcott, 1975). The researcher interviews, observes, and collects materials. Reflexivity is our means of developing ourselves as information gatherers, of assessing ourselves as information gatherers, and of assuring our constituencies that we are providing information that is as balanced, inclusive, dispassionate, impartial, disinterested, and equitable as our purposes, questions, and theoretical frameworks permit. However, the process is always limited by individuals' capacities for introspection, by resources such as time and training, and by conventional expectations of the Spock-like scientist, all rationality and no feeling.

Reflexivity, Recursivity, and Reflectivity

Reflexivity is related to and often overlapping with reflectivity and recursivity, two other key tenants of qualitative methods and design. Recursivity supports our efforts to be reflexive, but we conceptualize it as a somewhat different process. Recursivity is working back and forth among research question, selection, collection, and analysis in a spiraling process whereby each decision made prompts the researcher to reconsider each previous decision for whether it should be changed. Researchers may also draw from multiple cognitive approaches—induction, deduction, abduction, narrative—to build arguments and substantiate claims, and they work back and forth among these throughout the inquiry process.

One example of recursivity in ordinary activity occurs in writing. As we write succeeding sentences, we review previous sentences to check whether they need changing in light of the material we have added. Just as recursivity contributes to effective writing, it contributes to effective qualitative research design. Recursive practice can be compared to linear practice where steps in a process are sequential and invariant and where decisions once made cannot be unmade or to haphazard practice where no order obtains at all. Of course, most of our actual practices are some blend of these—linear, recursive, and haphazard or serendipitous.

Recursivity can contribute to reflexivity if the researcher documents the recursive process and examines it alone or with assistance from others for evidence of imbalance, exclusion, inequity, partiality, hidden agendas, and tacit assumptions and presuppositions. However, recursiveness can be conducted un-self-consciously, with no attention to the doer and how it is done. In these cases recursivity likely contributes nothing to reflexivity.

In contrast we do not think that reflexivity can be quite so distinguished from the second process of reflectivity. Indeed, many qualitative methodologists might argue that they cannot be definitively separated. When we suggest that most qualitative traditions are reflective, what we mean is that qualitative research requires its practitioners to reflect throughout the entire process about their practice; it entails much more than learning a set of tools or techniques. Practicing research and conceptualizing research are not only integrated but also are interdependent facets of a holistic experience. Consequently, researchers must look broadly across human inquiry to find ideas and assumptions to match what they are perceiving. Often this reflection takes researchers into interdisciplinary terrain as we seek out and apply a variety of theoretical, conceptual, philosophical approaches in our studies. Reflective researchers may think broadly or narrowly to make sense of their data and activity, but they are more likely than not to cross disciplinary boundaries in pursuing this sense making. Whether they reflect on themselves as the instruments, doers, conductors of their studies, however, varies. We may reflect on our practices without specifically considering ourselves as practitioners. We believe that this quality is best formulated as multiple continua. Creative research requires thoughtfulness so most researchers are required to be reflective, but may differ in the degree to which they reflect and what they reflect about. We may be more or less reflective about techniques of data selection, collection, and analysis, about overall design issues, about the contexts and people we study, about the theories and concepts that frame our research questions, and about ourselves as research workers. Researchers can be reflective without being reflexive, but reflexivity requires reflection.

Formulating the Reflexive-Reflective Relationship

Figure 9.1, "Human Frameworks," is one conceptual mapping of the reflexive-reflective endeavor that we have found useful in teaching. All scholars have personal and cultural histories and disciplinary experiences and knowledge, and many also have histories and experiences of vocational and avocational practices. We are children of particular families, members of specific cultural groups, participants in varieties of work and play activities, and students of academic fields. The personal and cultural experiences on the left of the graphic inform our reflexivity while the practitioner and disciplinary experiences on the right inform our reflectivity. In reality these are all intertwined and intermeshed, but we separate them here to articulate what they are. We bring these four areas of experience, knowledge, and presuppositions into any research project. In the figure we represent this in the center of the graphic. The frameworks we bring to our research are composed in part of underlying assumptions about values, knowledge, and reality. These influence the questions we pose about the world. Our contention is that all scholarly research poses questions about both how the world *is* and how the world *could be*: How does the world work as we find it and how could it work differently with the appropriate intervention? These are the categories commonly labeled basic and applied research, but we believe most research has aspects of both dimensions. Finally, scholars emerge from research studies with different understandings, experiences, and assumptions than those they had initially. With careful consideration we learn to formulate our personal history as standpoints, our cultural history as worldviews, our practitioner experiences as pedagogies, and our disciplinary experiences as developing theories. Over time as we begin and end research projects, our frameworks change and develop—sometimes consistently, but at

Figure 9.1: Human Frameworks

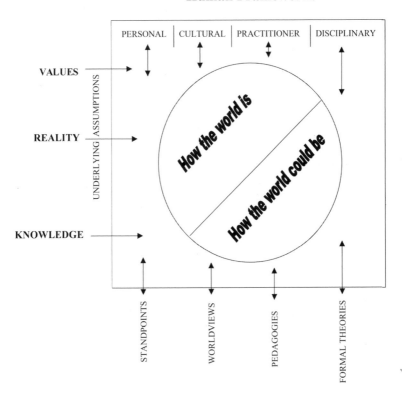

other times we may abandon dead ends, reverse direction, or even transform the direction of our work entirely.

We use Figure 9.1 to aid students, colleagues, and ourselves in mapping where we have been, what we are doing now, and how we might proceed in the future. It helps us sort out the challenges we face in proceeding reflexively.

Reflexive Challenges

Being reflexive requires us to be self-conscious. We must attend to ourselves as decision makers, agents, and actors. First, given that maturity and expertness partly depend on becoming un-self-conscious about much of what we do so that we can focus on the task at hand (see Benner, 1984; Dreyfus & Dreyfus, 1986), this can be a difficult process. We have to unlearn both the skill of and the desire for living un-self-consciously. Drawing on our adolescent selves may be one way of achieving this: remembering how to think about the performance of our lives and how it is perceived by others. Second, to the degree that the focus of our research is others and not ourselves, this self-consciousness may tempt us to self-absorption when we most need to be attentive to our participants. This is one of the many balancing acts that qualitative researchers face. We can overfocus on ourselves doing the research to the point that we lose our questions and our relationships with participants. Separating by time, place, and materials our reflections on self from reflections on participants may help address this issue. Third, disclosing our subjectivities through reflexivity may open us to charges of bias, prejudice, and being unscientific that other researchers, more discrete about their roles and conduct, may avoid. How much a researcher discloses and to what audiences is a judgment to be made, and it depends on context and purpose (see Passoth & Rowland, 2013, for an account of one such endeavor in disclosure).

Becoming Reflexive

So how do we prepare our students and our selves to become reflexive, to practice reflexivity, and to improve this practice? The following are the topics we address and the questions we pose to each other and that we expect our students to consider and reconsider throughout their research programs.

1. Know who you are. What personal history, experiences, skills and knowledge do you bring to research and inquiry? What are your values and ethics? What can you do? What can't you do? How do your temperament and personality influence how you view yourself, others, the world? What social and cultural identities affect your views of the world? As instruments we must first know ourselves, our strengths, and our limitations.

2. Know what and how you know and learn. What are your assumptions and presuppositions about knowledge and learning? Figure out your epistemology. This is what underlies your instrumentality.

3. Substantiate and corroborate by documenting your experience throughout the research. Keep a research journal where you record your thinking, decisions, actions, and feelings about the research process. For decisions you make, what alternatives do you have? What do you choose and why? Who and what are influencing you? You use this record to build a research autobiography at some point. Make the record as complete as possible but still doable. Select a format, media, and timing that fit how you work. Audio records work for some, computer diaries for others; some of us keep our records on handy slips of paper and stash them in manila folders—dated, so we know when we wrote them.

4. Read, view, search. Read specifically in your topical and methodological areas, but also read widely. In her qualitative methods book, Delamont (1992) recommends reading fiction, poetry, and nonfiction unrelated to our research as a strategy to open up our analytic imaginations to concepts and images we might not otherwise have considered. Likewise, seeking direct and vicarious experiences through art, recreation, and reading challenges us to formulate ourselves in relation to others and their creations. It heightens our senses of who we are and who we are not.

5. Compare yourself with others. Humans live in social worlds, and our identities are relational. How is your study like those of others and different from those of others? How much of the difference is due to the personal experience and history you bring to your research? We are not so much interested in comparisons of quality here but comparisons that allow us to know ourselves better by how we are like others and different from others. Comparisons of quality should, of course, be addressed, but focused on strengths and limitations. Part of knowing ourselves is knowing the value of our productions relative to those of others.

6. Open yourself to others' critique: be vulnerable. Knowledge is created by human learning. It begins in "not knowing" or ignorance. Letting ourselves "not know" makes us vulnerable. Likewise, sharing candidly our journeys from ignorance

to knowledge, how we went about addressing our questions, makes us vulnerable. The more we reveal about our processes, the more we expose to critique, as Passoth and Rowland (2013) document. However, not disclosing has its own consequences. People cannot assess the strengths and limitations of the results of research without knowing how the research was conducted. Although some may seize on our limitations to dismiss our work, most fellow researchers are disarmed when we are able to identify the limitations for them. So be bold and self-assess and self-critique.

Conclusion

Reflexivity is one of the more challenging processes of qualitative design. It can leave us nowhere to hide. It can also provide us with the respect and admiration of our colleagues. It requires a research life style that is open, flexible, and candid. It requires strength of character, confidence in identity(ies), and attention to how we live our research projects, and we assert that reflexivity results in a mindful life style.

References

Benner, P. (1984). *From novice to expert: Excellence and power in clinical nursing practice*. Menlo Park, CA: Addison-Wesley.

Delamont, S. (1992). *Fieldwork in educational settings: Methods, pitfalls, and perspectives*. London: Falmer Press.

DeMarrais, K. B. (1998). *Inside stories: Qualitative research reflections*. Mahwah, NJ: Lawrence Erlbaum.

Dreyfus, H. L, & Dreyfus, S. E. (1986). *Mind over machine: The power of human intuition and expertise in the era of the computer*. New York: The Free Press.

Passoth, J. -H., & Rowland, N. J. (2013). Beware of allies! Notes on analytical hygiene in actor-network account-making. *Qualitative Sociology, 36*, 465–483.

Preissle, J. (2008). Subjectivity Statement. In L. M. Given (Ed.),*The Sage encyclopedia of qualitative research methods* (Vol. 2, pp. 844–845). Thousand Oaks, CA: Sage.

Wolcott, Harry F. (1975). Criteria for an ethnographic approach to research in schools. *Human Organization, 34*, 111–127.

Chapter 10

Coda

The Death of Data?[1]

Norman K. Denzin

Data Are Dead. Data died a long time ago, but few noticed. Poststructuralism took away positivism's claim to a God's eye view of the world, that view which said objective observers could turn the world and its happenings into things that could be turned into data (Richardson, 2000, p. 928; St. Pierre & Adams, 2011, p. 620). The argument was straight forward, things, words, "become data only when theory acknowledges them as data" (St. Pierre & Adams, 2011, p. 621). In a single gesture, doubt replaces certainty, no theory, method, discourse, genre, or tradition has "a universal and general claim as the 'right' or privileged form of authoritative knowledge" (St. Pierre & Pillow, 2000, p. 928). Indeed all claims to universal truth "mask particular interests in local, cultural, and political struggles" (Richardson, 2000, p. 928).

Data Died a Long Time Ago. Who noticed? Science-(and evidence-) based research initiatives (SBR; EBR) keep the word in the limelight. Mixed methods is the new watchword, an old strategy which says data can be both qualitative and quantitative.[2] By keeping a focus on data, and its management, traditional qualitative inquiry

From Denzin, Norman K. 2013. *Cultural Studies ↔ Critical Methodologies,* *13*(4), 353–356 © SAGE Publications. Republished in *Qualitative Inquiry and the Politics of Research* edited by Norman K. Denzin and Michael D. Giardina, 197–206. (Left Coast Press, Inc., 2015). All rights reserved.

texts are also complicit in this conversation. Complicit, too, are those who call for the use of computer assisted qualitative data analysis software (CAQDAS) (see Davidson & di Gregorio, 2011, p. 627).

Data Are Alive and Well. The skeptics will not be quieted. The practices that produce data remain under assault. Criticism comes from all sides, from the new materialisms to decolonizing, feminist, critical, sacred, queer, Asian, postempirical, postqualitative, and posthumanist pedagogies (see Denzin, 2010, 2012; Jackson & Mazzei, 2009, 2012; Koro-Ljungberg, 2010; Lather, 2007; Lincoln, Lynham & Guba, 2011; MacLure, 2003, 2011, 2012; Richardson, 2000; Smith, 2012; St. Pierre & Adams, 2011; St. Pierre, Adams & Pillow, 2000).

Where Do Data Live? Ostensibly, data would have no place in these left pole epistemologies;[3] after all, they offer harsh criticisms of conventional, traditional qualitative methodology. Ironically, such has not been the case. The dreaded word keeps resurfacing, still hanging around, even in deconstructionist discourse. Here is a sampling of phrases found in recent works:

- think with data
- practice plugging theory and data into one another
- use transgressive data
- stay close to the data
- code data, decode data, deconstruct data.

So is the word still alive, or alive but with a different set of meanings?

A Rupture

More is at play. There is a rupture that goes beyond data and their meanings. The traditional concepts of narrative, meaning, voice, presence, and representation are also put under erasure, regarded as pernicious "left-overs" from the twin ruins of postpositivism and humanistic qualitative inquiry (Jackson & Mazzei, 2012, p. vii; St Pierre & Pillow, 2000). Materialist feminist ontologies, inspire new analytics of data analysis, including defractive readings of data (Jackson & Mazzei, 2012). Postmethodologists, posthumanist, postempirical, and postqualitative frameworks call for new models of science, second empiricisms, reimagined social sciences, capacious sciences, sciences of difference, a science defined by becoming, a double(d) science (Lather, 2007; MacLure, 2011; St. Pierre & Adams, 2011, p. 613). Where do data fit in these new spaces? Is there any longer even a need for the word? Why keep the word after you have deconstructed it?

At the same time, in some other wilderness a radical middle based on social justice and transformational politics engages these competing voices. Hoping to make some sense out of everything after having already gotten lost once before (Lather, 2007).

▓

It is clear that a great deal is happening. We are beyond the arguments of even ten years ago. Critics are united by commitments to social justice. The arguments for and against data (new or old versions) are debated, new places are sought.

Whither Data. For some, this is a place where there are no data, where the search is for justice, moral arguments, a politics of representation which seeks utopias of possibility, a politics of hope not a politics based on data (Madison, 2010). For others data are reconfigured, reread through new ontologies and new interpretive analytics (St. Pierre & Adams, 2011). For others data are used for practical purposes, in framing claims for changes in social policy (Gomez, Puigvert & Flecha, 2011).

These reconfigurations move in three directions at the same time. They interrogate the practices and politics of evidence that produce data. They support the call for new ways of making the mundane, taken-for-granted everyday world visible, whether through performance, or through disruptive postempirical methodologies. These unruly methodologies read and interrupt traces of presence, whether from film, recordings, or transcriptions. They do not privilege presence, voice, meaning, or intentionality. Rather, they seek performative interventions and representations that heighten critical reflective awareness leading to concrete forms of praxis.

Underneath it all it is assumed that we make the world visible through our interpretive practices. All texts have a material presence in the world. Nothing stands outside the text, even as it makes the material present. Neither the material nor the discursive is privileged. They fold into one another, get tangled up in one another. How a thing gets inside the text is shaped by a politics of representation. Language and speech do not mirror experience. They create experience, and in the process transform and defer that which is being described. Meanings are always in motion, incomplete, partial, contradictory. There can never be a final, accurate, complete representation of a thing, an utterance, or an action. There are only different representations of different representations. There is no longer any pure presence, description becomes inscription becomes performance.

Who Died? Qualitative inquiry under a postpositivist paradigm is dead, or should at least be placed in brackets. We seek a new paradigm, one which doubles back on its self and wanders in spaces that have not yet been named (Lather, 2007; St. Pierre & Adams, 2011).

The Politics of Evidence[4]

In this new terrain it is understood that data and evidence are never morally or ethically neutral. Paraphrasing Morse (2006, pp. 415–416), who quotes Larner (2004, p. 20), the politics and political economy of evidence, also known as data, is not a question of evidence or no evidence. It is rather a question of who has the power to control the definition of evidence, who defines the kinds of materials that count as evidence, who determines what methods best produce the best forms of evidence, whose criteria and standards are used to evaluate quality evidence. The politics of data, the politics of evidence, cannot be separated from the ethics of evidence.

Data as Evidence. How is evidence turned into data? This is not a simple process, and not accomplished by waving a wand over a body of observations, or plugging observations into a theory. Nor is there a detailed discussion of how data are to be used to produce generalizations, test and refine theory, and permit causal reasoning. And here, the fog of postpositivism lingers. It is clear, though, that as data become a commodity they carry the weight of the scientific process (see Charmaz, 2005; Maxwell, 2004).

Data's Voice. Data are never silent, they speak up, get rowdy, act up, resist being turned into commodities, produced by researchers, perhaps owned by the government, or by funding agencies, or by researchers. Data resist being shared. Data want agency. Data want to determine their own meanings. Data do not want to be owned, nor shared.

The injunction to engage in data sharing requires amplification. Data sharing involves complex moral considerations that go beyond sending a body of coded data to a colleague. Money, and concerns for auditing from the audit culture, seem to drive the process. This is evidenced in the emphasis placed on quality peer reviews. If quality data can be produced and shared, then granting agencies get more science for less money. Quality projects need to be funded. For this to happen granting agencies need quality reviewers who are using stable rating systems.

But the peer-review system is not immune to political influence. Kaplan (2004) has demonstrated that in the United States, the Bush Administration systematically stacked federal advisory and peer-review committees with researchers whose views matched the president's on issues ranging from stem-cell research to ergonomics, faith-based science, AIDS, sex education, family values, global warming, and environmental issues in public parks.

Data Will Not Die

Like those nineteenth century vampires that would not die, positivism's data cannot be killed. The movements that keep data alive will not wither away under postempirical, post-materialist, non-representational poststructural attacks. Rather, like Bram Stoker's (1897) Dracula, attacks seem to make the forces for data grow stronger. This is especially so for those who valorize such terms as method, epistemology, evidence, reliability, and validity.

Data as Vampire. It appears, as with Stoker's Dracula, that data, the very word, invokes the anxieties of an age. Of course data's fears are not the fears of Stoker's late Victorian patriarchy. Data's fears, rather, are those of a twenty-first century neoliberal audit culture anchored in a postpositivism that will not go away. Of course there is nowhere to go if the world cannot be turned into data.

Fifteen Reasons for Not Using the Word 'Data,' or, All the Things Data Can't Do

1. The word data invokes a positivist epistemology and a politics of evidence based on terms like reliability and validity;
2. The word data invokes a positivist ontology which turns the world into nouns and other things;
3. The word data turns things into commodities that can be counted and sold;
4. The word data perpetuates the myth that objective observers can make the world visible through their methodological practices;
5. Data are not things that can be collected, coded or analyzed; data are processes constructed by the researcher's interpretive practices;
6. Data have agency; they are not passive;
7. Data have had their day;
8. Data are ideological productions;
9. Data are the handmaidens of an audit culture;
10. Data cannot speak;
11. Data cannot be plugged in;
12. Data are too messy for positivists;
13. Real data cannot be quantified;
14. The word data should be outlawed; replaced by what William James terms empirical materials;
15. Data are dead.
    15a. If you speak the word 'data' you have to sit in a corner and wear the black D Hat, also known as the Data Dunce Hat.

New Rules to Live By[5]

If we are to move forward positively, to get out of these data mine-fields, we must create a new narrative, a narrative of passion, and commitment, a narrative which teaches others that ways of know-ing are always already partial, moral, and political. This narrative will allow us to put our practices in proper perspective. Here are some of the certain things we can build our new practices around:

1. We have an ample supply of methodological rules and inter-pretive guidelines.

2. They are open to change and to differing interpretation, and this is how it should be.

3. There is no longer a single gold standard for qualitative work.

4. We value open-peer reviews in our journals.

5. Our empirical materials are performative. They are not com-modities to be bought, sold, and consumed.

6. Our feminist, communitarian ethics are not governed by IRBs.

7. Our science is open-ended, unruly, disruptive (MacLure, 2006; Stronach, Garratt, Pearce & Piper, 2007, p. 197).

8. Inquiry is always political and moral.

9. Objectivity and evidence are political and ethical terms.

A World Without Data

We live in a depressing historical moment, violent spaces, unend-ing wars against persons of color, repression, the falsification of evidence, the collapse of critical, democratic discourse, repres-sive neoliberalism, disguised as dispassionate objectivity, prevails. Global efforts to impose a new orthodoxy on critical social science inquiry must be resisted. A hegemonic politics of evidence cannot be allowed. Too much is at stake.

Imagine a world without data, a world without method, a world not run by auditors and postpositivists. A world where no one counts data and data no longer count. Imagine a world where research is no longer a dirty word (Smith, 2012, p. 1), a world without coding schemes, a world without computer software programs to analyze qualitative data, a world where utopian dreams are paramount, a world where we all work for a new politics of possibility (Madison, 2010). Just imagine.

Notes

1 This chapter was originally published under the same title in *Cultural Studies ↔ Critical Methodologies, 13*(4), 353–356. Reprinted with permission.
2 This is not the radical mixed methods middle outlined by Onwuegbuzie (2012).
3 See Eisenhart and Jurow (2011) on right pole (traditional) and left pole (poststructural) epistemologies.
4 The following section draws on Denzin (2009, pp. 62, 66–67).
5 This section borrows from Denzin (2011, p. 654).

References

Charmaz, K. (2005). Grounded theory in the 21st century: A qualitative method for advancing social justice research. In N. K. Denzin & Y. S. Lincoln (Eds.), *Handbook of qualitative research, 3/e* (pp. 507–535). Thousand Oaks, CA: Sage.

Davidson, J., & di Gregoria, S. (2011). Qualitative research and technology in the midst of a revolution. In N. K. Denzin & Y. S. Lincoln (Eds.), *Handbook of qualitative research, 4/e* (pp. 627–643). Thousand Oaks, CA: Sage.

Denzin, N. K. (2010). *The qualitative manifesto: A call to arms.* Walnut Creek, CA: Left Coast Press, Inc.

Denzin, N. K. (2012). The politics of evidence. In N. K. Denzin & Y. S. Lincoln (Eds.), *Handbook of qualitative research, 4/e* (pp. 645–659). Thousand Oaks, CA: Sage.

Eisenhart, M., & Jurow, A. S. (2011). Teaching qualitative research. In N. K. Denzin & Y. S. Lincoln (Eds.), *Handbook of qualitative research, 4/e* (pp. 699–714). Thousand Oaks, CA: Sage.

Gomez, A., Puigvert, L., & Flecha, R. (2011). Critical communicative methodology: Informing real social transformation through social research. *Qualitative Inquiry, 17,* 235–246.

Jackson, A. Y., & Mazzei, L. A. (2009). *Voice in qualitative inquiry: Challenging conventional, interpretive, and critical conceptions in qualitative research.* London: Routledge.

Jackson, A. Y., & Mazzei, L. A. (2012). *Thinking with theory in qualitative research: Viewing data across multiple perspectives.* London: Routledge.

Kaplan, E. (2004). *With God on their side: How Christian fundamentalists trampled science, policy, and democracy in the George Bush's White House.* New York: The New Press.

Koro-Ljungberg, M. (2010). Validity, responsibility and apora. *Qualitative Inquiry, 16,* 603–610.

Larner, G. (2004). "Family therapy and the politics of evidence." *Journal of Family Therapy, 26,* 17.

Lather, P. (2007). *Getting lost: Feminist efforts toward a double (d) science.* Albany, NY: SUNY Press.

Lincoln, Y. S., Lynham, S. A., & Guba, E. G. (2011). Paradigmatic controversies, contradictions, and emerging confluences, revisited. In N. K. Denzin & Y. S. Lincoln (Eds.), *Handbook of qualitative research, 4/e* (pp. 97–128). Thousand Oaks, CA: Sage.

MacLure, M. (2003). *Discourse in educational and social research.* Milton Keynes, UK: Open University.

MacLure, M. (2006). The bone in the throat: Some uncertain thoughts on baroque method. *International Journal of Qualitative Studies in Education, 19,* 729–746.

MacLure, M. (2011). Qualitative inquiry: Where are the ruins?" *Qualitative Inquiry, 17,* 997–1005.

MacLure, M. (2012). *The death of data?* Retrieved from www.esriblog.info/the-deaet-of-data/

Madison, D. S. (2010). Acts of activism: Human rights as radical performance. Cambridge, MA: Cambridge University Press.

Maxwell, J. A. (2004). Reemergent scientism, postmodernism, and dialogue across differences. *Qualitative Inquiry, 10,* 35–41.

Morse, J. M. (2006). Reconceptualizing qualitative inquiry. *Qualitative Health Research, 16,* 415–422.

Onwuegbuzie, A. I. (2012). "Introduction: Putting the MIXED back into quantitative and qualitative research in educational research and beyond: Moving toward the radical middle." *International Journal of Multiple Research Approaches, 6,* 192–219.

Richardson, L. (2000). Writing: A method of inquiry. In N. K. Denzin & Y. S. Lincoln (Eds.), *Handbook of qualitative research, 2/e* (pp. 923–948). Thousand Oaks, CA: Sage.

Smith, L. T. (2012). *Decolonizing methodologies: Research and indigenous peoples, 2/e*. London: Zed Books.

St. Pierre,, E. A. (2011). Post qualitative research: The critique and the coming after. In N. K. Denzin & Y. S. Lincoln (Eds.), *Handbook of qualitative research, 4/e* (pp. 611-626). Thousand Oaks, CA: Sage.

St. Pierre, E. A., & Pillow, W. (Eds.). (2000). *Working the ruins: Feminist poststructural methods in education*. New York: Routledge.

Stoker, B. (1897). *Dracula*. London: Archibald Constable.

Stronach, I., Garratt, D., Pearce, C., & Piper, H. (2007). Reflexivity, the picturing of selves, the forging of method. *Qualitative Inquiry, 13*, 179–203.

Index

About the Editors and Authors

Editors

Norman K. Denzin is Distinguished Professor of Communications, College of Communications Scholar, and Research Professor of Communications, Sociology, and Humanities at the University of Illinois, Urbana-Champaign. One of the world's foremost authorities on qualitative research and cultural criticism, Denzin is the author or editor of more than two dozen books, including *The Qualitative Manifesto*; *Qualitative Inquiry Under Fire*; *Reading Race*; *Interpretive Ethnography*; *The Cinematic Society*; *The Voyeur's Gaze*; and *The Alcoholic Self*. He is past editor of *The Sociological Quarterly*, co-editor (with Yvonna S. Lincoln) of four editions of the landmark *Handbook of Qualitative Research*, co-editor (with Michael D. Giardina) of ten plenary volumes from the annual International Congress of Qualitative Inquiry, co-editor (with Giardina) of *Qualitative Inquiry—Past, Present, & Future: A Critical Reader*, co-editor (with Lincoln) of the methods journal *Qualitative Inquiry*, founding editor of *Cultural Studies ↔ Critical Methodologies* and *International Review of Qualitative Research*, editor of three book series, and founding director of the International Congress of Qualitative Inquiry.

Michael D. Giardina is an Associate Professor of Sport, Culture, and Politics and Associate Director of the Center for Sport, Health, and Equitable Development at Florida State University. He is the author of *Sport, Spectacle, and NASCAR Nation: Consumption and the Cultural Politics of Neoliberalism* (Palgrave, 2011, with Joshua Newman), which received the 2012 Outstanding Book Award from the North American Society for the Sociology of Sport (NASSS) and was named to the 2012 *CHOICE* Outstanding Academic Titles list, and *Sporting Pedagogies: Performing Culture & Identity in the Global Arena* (Peter Lang, 2005), which received the 2006 Outstanding Book Award from NASSS. He is also the editor or co-editor of more than a dozen books on qualitative inquiry, cultural studies, and interpretive research, including most recently *Qualitative Inquiry—Past, Present, & Future: A Critical Reader* (with Norman K. Denzin; Left Coast Press, 2015). He is editor of the *Sociology of Sport Journal*, Special Issue Editor of *Cultural Studies ↔ Critical Methodologies*, and the associate director of the International Congress of Qualitative Inquiry.

Authors

Bryant Keith Alexander is Dean of the College Communication and Fine Arts and Professor of Communication Studies at Loyola Marymount University. He is an active scholar, lecturer and performer with publications in leading journals—along with major contributions in such volumes as the *Handbook of Critical and Indigenous Methodologies,* the *Handbook of Performance Studies,* the *Handbook of Qualitative Research (3/e);* the *Handbook of Communication and Instruction, the Handbook of Critical Intercultural Communication,* and the *Handbook of Autoethnography.* He is the co-editor of *Performance Theories in Education: Power, Pedagogy and the Politics of Identity* (2005), and author of *Performing Black Masculinity: Race, Culture, and Queer Identity* (2006) and *The Performative Sustainability of Race: Reflections on Black Culture and the Politics of Identity* (2012).

Laura Atkins is a doctoral candidate in the Department of Sociology at the University of Illinois, where she holds an appointment with ATLAS (Applied Technologies for Learning in the Arts and Sciences). Her dissertation research explores the psychosocial effects caused by toxic contamination within disease cluster communities.

David Lee Carlson is an Associate Professor in the Division of Teacher Education at Arizona State University. He focuses primarily on the importance of critical and queer theory in education, specifically the works of Michel Foucault, Pierre Bourdieu, and Jacque Derrida. His most current work explores the pedagogies of friendship and how they interact with gender and sexuality studies in education. He is the author of *Composing a Care of the Self: A Critical History of Writing Assessment in Secondary English Education* (Sense), and is currently working on two book projects. They include *(Re) Reading Queer Theory: The Grammar of Recognition and the Pedagogies of Friendship (*Sense) and *Foucault and Bourdieu in Conversation* (Sense). He is also collecting life histories of gay men in the southwestern part of the United States as a way to generate a sense of history of LGBTQ people in this region. He was the 2012 recipient of the Promising Research Scholar award by Mary Lou Fulton Teachers College at Arizona State University.

Elliot P. Douglas is Associate Professor of Materials Science and Engineering, Dean's Fellow for Engineering Education, and Distinguished Teaching Scholar at the University of Florida. His research interests are in the areas of active learning pedagogies, problem-solving, critical thinking, diversity in engineering, and qualitative methodologies.

Kathleen deMarrais is Professor and Department Head of the Department of Lifelong Learning, Administration, and Policy, and former Associate Dean for Academic Programs, at the University of Georgia. She is the author or editor of numerous books, including *Foundations for Research: Methods of Inquiry in Education and the Social Sciences* (with Stephen Lapan; Routledge, 2003), *The Way Schools Work: A Sociological Analysis* (1999; Longman), and *Qualitative Pedagogy* (with Judith Preissle; Routledge, forthcoming).

Uwe Flick is Professor for Qualitative Social and Educational Research at the Free University of Berlin. Before that he worked at the Alice Salomon University in Berlin in the field of health services research, still his major area of research, with a focus on vulnerability and service utilization. He is author or editor of numerous textbooks and handbooks, most of which have been translated in several languages in Europe, Latin America, and

Asia. Books include *An Introduction to Qualitative Research* (5th ed. 2014, SAGE), *The SAGE Handbook of Qualitative Data Analysis* (2014, SAGE), *Introducing Research Methodology—A Beginners' Guide to Doing a Research Project* (2nd ed. 2015, SAGE), and the *Qualitative Research Kit* (2007, 8 Volumes, SAGE).

Mirka Koro-Ljungberg is Professor of Qualitative Research at the Arizona State University. Her research and publications focus on various conceptual and theoretical aspects of qualitative inquiry and participant-driven methodologies. In particular, her scholarship brings together theory and practice, the promotion of epistemology, and the development of situated and experimental methodologies.

Patti Lather is Emeritus Professor in the School of Education Policy and Leadership at Ohio State University. She is the author of four books, *Getting Smart: Feminist Research and Pedagogy With/in the Postmodern* (1991 Critics Choice Award), *Troubling the Angels: Women Living with HIV/AIDS* (co-authored with Chris Smithies; 1998 *CHOICE* Outstanding Academic Title), *Getting Lost: Feminist Efforts Toward a Double(d) Science* (2008 Critics Choice Award), and *Engaging (Social) Science: Policy from the Side of the Messy* (2010, 2011 Critics Choice Award). She is a 2009 inductee of the American Educational Research Association (AERA) Fellows.

Patrick Lewis is Associate Professor of Early Childhood Education at the University of Regina, Canada. He is interested in the relationship between play, art, and narrative, as well as other landscapes of critical inquiry. He is the author of *How We Think, But Not In Schools: A Storied Approach to Teaching* (Sense, 2009), and editor of *Challenges Bequeathed: Taking up the Challenges of Dwayne E. Huebner* (with J. Tupper, 2009; Sense).

Judith Preissle is Professor Emeritus of Lifelong Learning, Administration, and Policy at the University of Georgia, where she was a Distinguished Aderhold Professor. She has also been an AERA Fellow and, in 2014, she was the recipient of the Lifetime Achievement Award in Qualitative Inquiry from the International Congress of Qualitative Inquiry.

Elizabeth Adams St. Pierre is Professor and Graduate Coordinator of Language and Literacy Education at the University of Georgia. Her work has appeared in a range of scholarly journals, including *International Review of Qualitative Research, Educational Researcher, Qualitative Inquiry, Journal of Contemporary Ethnography*, and *International Journal of Qualitative Studies in Education*. She is also the editor of *Working the Ruins: Feminist Poststructural Theory and Methods in Education* (Routledge, 2000; with Wanda Pillow).

David J. Therriault is an Associate Professor in the School of Human Development and Organizational Studies in the College of Education at the University of Florida. He was formerly a Postdoctoral Fellow at Florida State University's Psychology Department, working with Dr. Rolf Zwaan from 2001 to 2004. His primary research interests include the representation of text in memory, comprehending time and space in language, the link between attention and intelligence, the use of perceptual symbols in language, creativity and problem solving, and educational issues related to these topics.

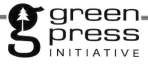
green press
INITIATIVE

Left Coast Press, Inc. is committed to preserving ancient forests and natural resources. We elected to print this title on 30% post consumer recycled paper, processed chlorine free. As a result, for this printing, we have saved:

5 Trees (40' tall and 6-8" diameter)
2 Million BTUs of Total Energy
380 Pounds of Greenhouse Gases
2,065 Gallons of Wastewater
138 Pounds of Solid Waste

Left Coast Press, Inc. made this paper choice because our printer, Thomson-Shore, Inc., is a member of Green Press Initiative, a nonprofit program dedicated to supporting authors, publishers, and suppliers in their efforts to reduce their use of fiber obtained from endangered forests.

For more information, visit www.greenpressinitiative.org

Environmental impact estimates were made using the Environmental Defense Paper Calculator. For more information visit: www.papercalculator.org.